The Native Ameri Herbalist's Bible 3

C000061197

• The Lost Book of Herbal Remedies •

The Ultimate Herbal Dispensatory to Discover the Secrets and Forgotten Practices of Native American Herbal Medicine

Linda Osceola Naranjo

Table of Contents

The Native American Herbalist's Bible 3 • 1

Introduction 2

Abscess and Gingivitis.. 4

    HERBAL MOUTHWASH.. 4

    SKIN-ABSCESS-FIGHTING TEA 5

    TOPICAL WASH FOR ABSCESSES AND GINGIVITIS 5

Acne.. 6

    SKIN TONER.. 6

    FACIAL STEAM.. 7

    ACNE-FIGHTING TEA 7

    ACNE WASH 8

Aging 9

    ANTI-AGING TEA 1 9

    ANTIAGING TEA 2 9

Allergies.. 10

    ALLERGY RELIEF TEA... 11

    QUICK ALLERGY TEA 11

    FLOWER DECOCTION 12

    NETTLE TEA.. 12

Anemia 13

    ANEMIA TEA 13

Arthritis 14

    ARTHRITIS MILDING TEA 14

    QUICK ANALGESIC ARTHRITIS TEA... 15

    NIGHTLY ARTHRITIS TEA.. 15

    ARTHRITIS OINTMENT 15

Asthma.. 16

    QUICK-ACTING ASTHMA TEA 16

    SOOTHING TEA 16

Back Pain 18

    SPINE'S FINE TINCTURE.. 18

    WARMING COMPRESS 19

    SCIATIC PAIN TEA 19

    ANALGESIC DAILY TEA FOR BACK PAIN... 20

    SOOTHING BACK PAIN TEA 20

Bedsores..21

   BEDSORE TOPICAL WASH 21

Bites and Stings..22

   COOLING COMPRESS...22

   BUG BITE RELIEF SPRAY..23

   TOPICAL WASH FOR BITES AND STINGS.............................23

   SKIN SOOTHING OINTMENT 23

Bronchitis..25

   FIRE CIDER 25

   THROAT-SOOTHING TEA 26

   SWEET SOOTHING TEA 26

Burns and Sunburns..28

   BURN-HEALING HONEY 28

   SUNBURN SPRAY..29

   BURN POULTICE 29

   IMMUNITY STRENGTHENER 30

Canker Sores..31

   ANTI-INFLAMMATORY MOUTHWASH 31

Cold Sores..32

   COLD SORE COMPRESS 32

   COLD SORE BALM 33

   COLD SORE TEA 33

   COLD SORE MOUTHWASH 33

Constipation...35

   BOWEL-HYDRATING INFUSION...35

   BOWEL-MOTIVATING TINCTURE 36

   BOWEL-SOOTHING TEA 36

   PURIFYING DIGESTIVE TEA 36

Cough and Cold..38

   LUNG-LUBRICATING TEA 39

   ANTITUSSIVE OXYMEL...39

   COUGH SYRUP 40

   SOOTHING COUGH AND COLD FORMULA 40

   LAKOTA COUGH AND COLD FORMULA.............................40

   LUMBEE COUGH AND COLD FORMULA.............................40

   QUICK-ACTING COUGH AND COLD FORMULA 41

EXPECTORATING COUGH AND COLD TEA...41

DECONGESTANT TEA...41

ANTITUSSIVE FLOWER TEA...42

QUICK-ACTING MULLEIN COUGH SYRUP...42

ELECAMPANE COUGH SYRUP...42

HOREHOUND LOZENGES...42

Cramps...44

MUSCLE-WARMING OINTMENT...44

MUSCLE CRAMP TEA...44

MUSCLE RUB...45

DIARRHEA...45

ASTRINGENT TEA...46

CINNAMON POWDER CAPSULES...46

QUICK AND EASY DIARRHEA TEA...47

SOOTHING DIARRHEA TEA...47

IROQUOIS TEA...47

Fatigue...49

SHAKE-IT-OFF FORMULA...49

UP-AND-ABOUT MORSELS...50

PICK-ME-UP TEA...50

INVIGORATING TEA...51

Fever...52

FEVER-INDUCING TEA...53

FEVER-BREAKING TEA...53

FEVER RELIEF TEA...54

QUICK-ACTING FEVER TEA...54

Food Intolerances...55

GUT-HEAL TEA...56

BUILD-UP BROTH...56

STOP-FLATULENCE TEA...57

COLON-SOOTHING TEA...57

QUICK-ACTING FLATULENCE TEA...58

GUT-CLEARING TEA...58

DAILY DIGESTIVE TEA...58

PEPPERY INDIGESTION TEA...58

Hangover...60

TAKE-IT-EASY NEXT DAY INFUSION...60

NO-FUSS HANGOVER TEA 61

QUICK-ACTING HANGOVER TEA 61

SPICY HANGOVER TEA 61

Headache 63

COOLING HEADACHE TEA 63

WARMING HEADACHE TEA 64

PEPPERY HEADACHE TEA 64

SOOTHING HEADACHE TEA 65

HEARTBURN/REFLUX/GERD 65

MARSHMALLOW INFUSION 66

PREVENTIVE BITTER TINCTURE 67

QUICK-ACTING HEARTBURN TEA 67

SOOTHING HEARTBURN TEA 67

Hypertension 68

SOFTHEARTED TEA 68

FREE-FLOWING CIRCULATION TEA 69

ANTI-CONGESTIVE TEA 69

ARTERIOSCLEROSIS PREVENTIVE TEA 69

Indigestion/Dyspepsia 71

PRE-EMPTIVE BITTER TINCTURE 71

CARMINATIVE TINCTURE 72

DIGESTIVE TEA 72

STRONG DIGESTIVE TEA 72

QUICK-ACTING DIGESTIVE TEA 73

Insomnia 74

END-OF-THE-DAY ELIXIR 74

SLEEP! FORMULA 75

INSOMNIA RELIEF TEA 75

SWEET DREAMS TEA 76

Menstrual cycle irregularities 77

STEADY CYCLE TEA 78

BLEED ON! TEA 78

DAILY SOOTHING MENSTRUAL TEA 79

DYSMENORRHEA TEA 79

CRAMP RELIEF TEA 79

Nausea and Vomiting 80

CALMING TEA 81

GINGER EMERGENCY FORMULA 81

Rash 83

DRY RASH SALVE 83

WEEPY RASH POULTICE..84

SKIN-SOOTHING TEA 84

RASH WASH 85

Sinusitis/Stuffy Nose 86

SINUS-CLEARING STEAM BATH..87

SINUS-RELIEVING TEA 87

MUCUS-FREEING TEA 88

Sore Throat 89

SORE THROAT TEA 89

HERBAL GARGLE 90

THROAT-SOOTHING TEA 91

FRUITY GARGLE 91

SWEET COUGH DROPS 91

Sprains and Strains 92

SOFT TISSUE INJURY LINIMENT 93

TOPICAL PAIN RELIEF 93

QUICK-ACTING PAIN RELIEF TEA 93

SWEET RELIEF TEA 94

Stress 95

RESCUE ELIXIR..95

SOOTHE UP! TEA..96

NERVE-SOOTHING TEA..97

CALM DOWN TEA 97

SHAKE-IT-OFF TEA 97

Wounds 98

WOUND WASH 98

PINE RESIN SALVE 99

TOPICAL APPLICATION FOR ABRASIONS 100

TOPICAL WASH FOR CUTS 100

Conclusion 101

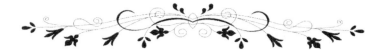

Introduction

We live in a country where the cure for virtually any disease and ailment is within our grasp. In our forests, meadows, plains, and gardens grow small, seemingly insignificant flowers and herbs, plants that we don't look twice at, and trees of which we don't even bother to learn the name. Yet, they are the key to a better, healthier, and more sustainable way of life.

Our forefathers, more attuned with nature that we could ever imagine to be, understood that and took carefully and sparingly the gifts that Nature offered to heal themselves and grow stronger. We have lost that knowledge. Only starting from the 1970s, a renewed interest in botanic medicine has uncovered the depth of the Native American knowledge of plants and their healing powers. The research has not only helped herbalists, but physicians and scientist as well that re-discovered substances that the Native Americans people knew about for hundreds of years.

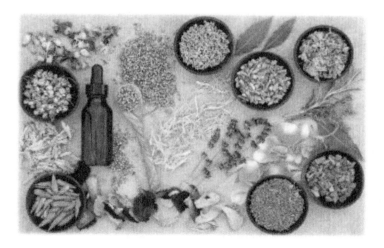

The mountains, I become a part of it...
The herbs, the fir tree, I become a part of it.
The morning mists, the clouds, the gathering waters,
I become a part of it.
The wilderness, the dew drops, the pollen...
I become a part of it.

Navajo Chant

You don't need to put at risk the delicate natural balance of your body by taking drugs and medications, if an easily available natural solution is just outside your door. Harvest carefully or grow your own herbs, learn to know your body and what works best for you, communicate with the nature surrounding you, and you will in a small way bring back a culture that for too long as been treated as inferior.

This book will teach how to find and treat the herbs the way the native American tribes did: from the forest to your herbalist table, but you will have to find your way to listen to your body and the plants around you.

To aid you in your holistic journey, we have decided to divide the book in three volumes. The first volume offers you a full theoretical approach to Native American medicine and the herbal medicines methods and preparations. The second volume is a complete encyclopedia of all the most relevant herbs used in traditional Native American medicine, complete with modern examples, doses, and where to find them, making it a very effective field guide. This third volume is a "recipe book" of sorts: it offers easy herbal solutions to the most common diseases a budding naturopath can encounter. It is meant as a jumping point to find your own way to treat yourself and your fellow man and will come in handy even to the most experienced herbalist.

Please keep in mind that, because herbs were the very first medicines, they can be very powerful. Do not gather herbs from the wild unless you know what you are doing. And please, grow your own herbs whenever possible; native herbs are becoming increasingly rare, and many are threatened with extinction.

Choosing the right herbs and herbal combinations for your health needs is most important for you. Follow three easy steps to identify and satisfy your herbal and nutritional needs:
1. Identify the injury or disorder that is affecting you.
2. Identify the areas of your health status and specific needs that require additional support.
3. Choose the most appropriate treatment program from this book that fits your needs. This should include herbs, enzymes, vitamins, minerals, and phytochemicals.

As always, if you are pregnant or nursing, if you suffer from a chronic condition such as heart disease or diabetes, or if you are currently taking medications of any kind, please consult with your physician or a well-trained herbal specialist before self-treating. Herbs and other supplements can alter the way your body utilizes other medicines. They can sometimes improve the efficacy of medicines and, at other times, interfere with the absorption or action of a particular drug.

If you have any questions about the appropriateness of any treatment, seek the services of a well-trained health-care professional. This book and the formulas contained herein are not intended to replace the services of a well-trained health-care professional.

Abscess and Gingivitis

An abscess is a local accumulation of pus. It can occur almost anywhere on or in the body, but it most frequently occurs on the skin and on the gums of the mouth. Abscesses can be very tender and painful and are marked by inflammation, swelling, heat, redness, and often fever. Abscesses are caused by an infection, so it is often treated with antibiotics. But herbs are an effective and safe alternative, without the side effects of antibiotics.

Relevant tissue states: heat (inflammation), dampness, laxity
Relevant herbal actions: anti-inflammatory, antimicrobial, astringent, vulnerary

Herbal Allies

- Barberries
- Calendula flower
- Chamomile flower
- Echinacea
- Goldenrod leaf and flower
- Licorice root
- Meadowsweet flower
- Oregon grape root
- Plantain leaf
- Rose
- Sage leaf
- Self-heal leaf and flower
- Thyme leaf
- Uva-ursi leaf
- White Oak
- Yarrow leaf and flower
- Yerba Mansa

It can be very painful to have an abscess—a fluid-filled blister or infection—in the mouth. Gingivitis is an inflammation of the gums that can lead to loose teeth. Resist the urge to poke and prod at the gums too much—if you make them bleed, bacteria can move deeper. Treat your gums gently! Antimicrobial, astringent, anti-inflammatory, and wound-healing herbs fight infection and restore healthy tissue.

HERBAL MOUTHWASH

Makes 8 fluid ounces (16 to 20 swishes)

While saltwater works well on its own, adding herbs makes it much more effective. Adjust the amounts of each herb according to taste. Swish with ¼ to ½ fluid ounce of mouthwash after brushing, and swish well, getting between the teeth and throughout the mouth, for 2 to 5 minutes.

4 fluid ounces water
1 teaspoon sea salt
1 fluid ounce tincture of uva-ursi
1 fluid ounce tincture of yarrow

½ fluid ounce tincture of calendula
½ fluid ounce tincture of plantain
½ fluid ounce tincture of self-heal
¼ fluid ounce tincture of licorice
¼ fluid ounce tincture of meadowsweet

1.In a jar with a lid, combine all the ingredients. Cover the jar, label it, and shake well. This is shelf stable.
2.Use this mouthwash every time you brush—twice a day is best.

SKIN~ABSCESS~FIGHTING TEA

30 drops echinacea tincture (See Part One for directions for tinctures.)
60 drops yerba mansa tincture
1 cup warm water

1. Combine all the ingredients.
2. Take up to five times per day to stimulate the immune system and help eliminate the infection.

TOPICAL WASH FOR ABSCESSES AND GINGIVITIS

1 to 2 teaspoons barberries
1 tablespoon white oak bark
1 teaspoon echinacea root
1 teaspoon granulated Oregon grape root
2 cups boiling water

1. Combine the herbs in a glass container.
2. Pour the boiling water over the herbs and soak for 3 to 4 hours; strain.
3. Use three times a day as a wash. If you are using this tea to treat a gum abscess, be sure to swish the liquid around in your mouth for several minutes before spitting it out.

Acne

Acne is an inflammatory skin condition that commonly affects adolescents (because of increased glandular activity during the teen years). Acne occurs when the sebaceous glands, which are located just beneath the skin, become inflamed. These glands secrete an oil called sebum, which acts to lubricate the skin. Acne results when the pores of the skin become clogged by the sebum. Acne can occur any time in life and may be due to allergies, high-sugar or high-fat diets, heredity, the use of oral contraceptives and other drugs (such as cortisone), hormone changes, and stress.

Relevant tissue states: heat (inflammation), dampness (oily)
Relevant herbal actions: anti-inflammatory, antimicrobial, astringent, circulatory stimulant, liver stimulant, lymphatic

Herbal Allies

- Burdock
- Calendula flower
- Chamomile flower
- Dandelion root
- Echinacea
- Elder
- Ginger root
- *Gingko Biloba*
- Ginseng
- Licorice
- Milk thistle seed
- Rose
- Sage leaf
- Self-heal leaf and flower
- St. John's wort leaf and flower
- Thyme leaf
- Yarrow leaf and flower
- White Willow Bark

To cope with chronic skin problems, it's important to treat the issue from both the inside and the outside. Topical applications (compresses, poultices, and steams) of astringent, anti-inflammatory, and antimicrobial herbs will clear and tone the skin directly. Internal preparations (tea, tincture, capsules) of liver-stimulating, circulatory-stimulant, and lymphatic herbs support the health and nourishment of skin tissue from beneath.

SKIN TONER

Makes 12 fluid ounces (90+ applications)

The acidity and probiotics from the vinegar combine with the astringency of the witch hazel and rose to gently but effectively tonify the skin, reducing blemishes and protecting against breakouts. Be consistent; results will begin to show after a few days to a week of use. This simple skin toner is a key part of Katja's vibrant skin protocol. (Though she's 44 years old, everyone thinks she's a decade younger.) If your skin is sensitive, reduce the amount of apple cider vinegar.

4 fluid ounces apple cider vinegar (preferably raw, unfiltered)
4 fluid ounces nonalcoholic witch hazel extract
4 fluid ounces rose water, or strong, well-strained rose petal infusion

1.In a small nonreactive bowl, stir together the vinegar, witch hazel, and rose water. This mixture is shelf stable. Store in an airtight container.
2.Apply this toner once a day after washing your face. If your skin tends toward dryness, rub a few drops of oil (rosehip or olive) into the skin afterward.
3.Apply this toner a second or third time during the day if your acne is persistent, but don't scrub too hard or use harsh soaps—just rinse gently with water first.

FACIAL STEAM

Makes 2 cups dried herb mix (4 to 8 steams)

For an active breakout, especially one that is oily, a steam is a great way to effectively deliver circulation-enhancing, inflammation-reducing, and bacteria-eliminating herbal action right into the pores.

½ cup dried chamomile flower
½ cup dried sage leaf
½ cup dried thyme leaf
½ cup dried yarrow leaf and flower
½ gallon water

1.In a small bowl, stir together the chamomile, sage, thyme, and yarrow. Store in an airtight container.
2.Clean your face with gentle soap and water.
3.Make and execute an herbal steam: In a medium pot over high heat, boil the water. Place the pot on a heat-proof surface, someplace where you can sit near it, and make a tent with a blanket or towel. Add ¼ to ½ cup of the herb mixture to the water. Position your face over the steam and remain there for 5 to 20 minutes. (Bring a tissue; the steam also clears your sinuses!)
4.Follow with spot applications of raw or herb-infused honey.

ACNE-FIGHTING TEA

1 cup Oregon grape root tea
50 drops yellow dock tincture

Combine the ingredients. Take up to one-third of the mixture three times daily.

ACNE WASH

1 cup horsetail tea
30 drops gotu kola tincture

Combine ingredients in a glass container with a lid. Use as much as needed to wash the skin, three times daily.

Aging

We all want to live to a ripe old age without looking a day over twenty-nine! Unfortunately, aging is a fact of life that occurs as the body's ability to function declines. The process of aging—marked by wrinkles, aching joints, fatigue, and loss or graying of hair—is accelerated by a poor diet, lack of exercise, excessive exposure to sunlight's ultraviolet rays, and lifestyle choices including smoking and drug use. These and other factors increase free-radical activity. Free radicals are highly unstable molecules that damage the cells' DNA and interfere with the cells' ability to function. A number of herbs function as antioxidants, which effectively eliminate free radicals.

Herbal Allies:
- Ginkgo biloba
- Ginger
- Parsley
- Milk thistle
- Black currants
- Elderberries
- Horsetail

ANTI-AGING TEA 1

½ cup Ginkgo biloba tea
½ cup ginseng tea

1. Combine the ingredients.
2. Take one-third of a cup three times daily.

Ginkgo is known to improve memory, while ginseng can boost energy levels.

ANTIAGING TEA 2

5 drops cayenne tincture
30 drops burdock tincture
15 drops goldenseal tincture
10 drops ginger root tincture
½ cup slippery elm tea (page 72)
1 cup warm water

1. Combine all ingredients.
2. Take 2 to 3 tablespoons three times per day to improve circulation.

Allergies

An allergy is a hypersensitive reaction to any of a number of substances. Allergies occur when the body's immune system malfunctions, going into "overdrive" to help protect the body from a substance it sees as foreign. Allergies are very common in the United States. In fact, more than one-third of all Americans suffer from an allergy of one type or another. Common symptoms include nasal congestion, coughing, watery eyes, sneezing, fatigue, and headaches. Some allergies may cause hives or an itchy rash. Severe allergies can cause the blood pressure to drop to dangerously low levels, leading to anaphylactic shock and death.

Hay fever is an acute type of allergy usually caused by airborne pollens. Trees and grasses are the typical culprits in this condition. Symptoms of hay fever include itchy eyes, mouth, and throat; watery eyes; sneezing; nasal discharge; and headaches.

Some people are allergic to molds, pollens, and dusts. Others react to certain foods such as wheat, milk, peanuts, eggs, or shellfish. Certain cosmetics or chemicals and even bee stings bring grief to many. The best way to treat an allergy is to avoid the offending substance. When that isn't possible, herbs can help check the watery eyes, nasal discharge, and coughing that occur with some allergies.

Relevant tissue states: heat (inflammation), laxity (of the mucous membranes)
Relevant herbal actions: antihistaminic, anti-inflammatory, kidney supportive, liver stimulant

Herbal Allies

- Agrimony
- All-heal leaf and flower
- Barberry Root
- Calendula flower
- Goldenrod leaf and flower
- Goldenseal
- Ground Ivy
- Marigold
- Milk thistle seed
- Mullein leaf
- Nettle leaf
- Oregon grape root
- Oxeye daisy
- Pearly everlasting flowers
- Plantain leaf
- Yerba sante

Allergic reactions to pollen, dust, or pets are primarily due to excessive histamine production, which ignites the inflammation underlying the runny nose, itchy eyes, and excessive phlegm. Histamine isn't all bad, though; it's a necessary part of sleep regulation, brain function, and even sexual response! Antihistaminic herbs are ideal because, while they help relieve allergy symptoms, they won't overshoot the mark and suppress histamine so much they cause adverse effects.

When trying to resolve allergies, we also must support the liver and kidneys. Among other things, the liver produces histaminase—an enzyme that breaks down histamine. So, when it's sluggish or overworked, histamine builds up and the inflammatory response worsens. The kidneys also help clear inflammatory instigators from the system, so giving them extra support helps reduce allergic symptoms.

ALLERGY RELIEF TEA

Makes about 3 to 4 cups dried herb mix (enough for 18 to 22 quarts of tea)

Nettle and goldenrod contain the antioxidant quercetin, which, according to a 2006 study by Shaik et al., stabilizes mast cells and prevents the release of histamine. Meanwhile, mullein supports the mucous membranes in the lungs and sinuses, reducing phlegm and mucus and quelling cough. Calendula and licorice improve liver function. Feel free to add some honey to your tea—especially if it's raw, local honey! Unfiltered honey helps reduce allergic response because it contains some pollen grains. Introducing these to the body through the oral route helps it become less reactive to them when you inhale pollen in the springtime.

1 cup dried nettle leaf (see Tips)
1 cup dried goldenrod leaf and flower
½ cup dried mullein leaf
½ cup dried calendula flower
½ to 1 cup marshmallow leaf (optional)
2 to 4 tablespoons dried licorice root

1. In a medium bowl, mix together all the herbs, including the marshmallow (if using, for a dry constitution). Store in an airtight container.
2. Make a long infusion: Prepare a kettle of boiling water. Measure 2 to 3 tablespoons of herbs per quart of water and place in a mason jar or French press. Pour in the boiling water, cover, and steep for 8 hours, or overnight.
3. Drink a quart or more every day, especially in the month before and during your personal peak allergy season. The earlier you start, the less you'll suffer.

TIP: Omit the nettle leaf and increase the goldenrod if you take blood-thinning pharmaceuticals.
TIP: Want a quick fix? No time for tea? The simple combination of freeze-dried nettle leaf capsules and milk thistle seed capsules offers quick relief from allergy. Choose a high-quality brand, and take 2 of each (with plenty of water) every 4 hours.

QUICK ALLERGY TEA

1 teaspoon barberry root
1 teaspoon Oregon grape root
1 cup water

1. Combine the herbs in a pan and cover with the water.
2. Bring to a boil. Reduce heat and simmer for 30 minutes. Strain.
3. Take one-third cup three times daily.

FLOWER DECOCTION

1 teaspoon oxeye daisy leaves
1 teaspoon pearly everlasting flowers
1 teaspoon yerba sante leaves
3 cups boiling water

1. Combine the herbs in a glass container and cover with the water; steep for 30 minutes; strain.
2. To use, take one-half to one cup every six hours.

NETTLE TEA

2 tablespoons nettle leaves
1 teaspoon Oregon grape root
2 cups boiling water

1. Combine all the herbs in a glass container and cover with the water; steep for 30 minutes; strain.
2. Take one-quarter cup three times a day.

Anemia

Anemia is a blood disorder marked by either red blood cells containing too little hemoglobin or too few red blood cells in the blood. (Hemoglobin is the protein in red blood cells that carries oxygen.) Anemia can have a number of causes, including alcoholism, excessive bleeding, illness, infections, poor bone marrow function, poor diet, and pregnancy. It is important to determine the cause of the anemia and treat the underlying condition.

Herbal Allies

- Barberry
- Oregon Grape Root
- Nettle

ANEMIA TEA

2 teaspoons barberry root
2 teaspoons Oregon grape root
4 tablespoons nettle leaves
2 cups cold water

1. Combine the herbs in a glass container.
2. Cover with the water.
3. Soak overnight.
4. Strain.
5. Take up to one-half cup three times daily.

Arthritis

There are two types of arthritis: rheumatoid arthritis and osteoarthritis. Rheumatoid arthritis (RA) is an autoimmune condition where the body sees itself as the enemy. The immune system's antibodies attack the joints and soft tissues, causing inflammation, pain, and gradual deterioration of the joint. RA can be a debilitating condition, especially when it occurs in young children.

Osteoarthritis is a degenerative disease, also called wear-and-tear arthritis. This form of arthritis affects many of us as we age. It occurs as the joints wear out over time. It usually starts in the joints of the hands and feet but eventually can affect even the larger joints of the body. Both rheumatoid arthritis and osteoarthritis can cause pain and stiffness.

In addition to the herbs listed below, other beneficial herbs for arthritis include bilberry, black currant, nettle, and vervain. The following treatments are effective for both osteoarthritis and rheumatoid arthritis.

Herbal Allies

- Balsam Bilberry
- Black Cohosh
- Black Currant
- Blue Vervain
- Cascara Sagrada
- Cayenne
- Chamomile
- Devil's Claw
- Feverfew
- Mullein
- Nettle
- Sarsaparilla
- White willow bark
- Wild Cherry
- Yucca

ARTHRITIS MILDING TEA

2 teaspoons devil's claw tuber
3 teaspoons white willow bark
1 teaspoon feverfew herb
2 teaspoons yucca root
2 teaspoons sarsaparilla root
3 cups cold water

1. Combine the herbs in a glass container and cover with the water.
2. Soak overnight.
3. Drain.
4. Take one-half cup three times daily.

QUICK ANALGESIC ARTHRITIS TEA

25 drops black cohosh tincture
90 drops wild cherry bark tincture
90 drops mullein tincture
1 cup warm water

1. Combine the above herbs in a glass container and cover with the water.
2. Take one-third of the mixture three times daily.

NIGHTLY ARTHRITIS TEA

1 teaspoon black cohosh root
1 teaspoon chamomile flowers
1 teaspoon cascara sagrada bark
2 cups water

1. Combine the above herbs in a glass container; cover with the water; stir thoroughly to combine.
2. Place 1½ teaspoons of the mixture in one cup boiling water; steep for 10 minutes; strain.
3. Take one cup in the evening, just before going to bed.

ARTHRITIS OINTMENT

1 pound petroleum jelly
1 tablespoon Canada balsam
2 tablespoons cayenne
2 tablespoons chamomile

1. Melt one pound of petroleum jelly in a double boiler.
2. Add herbs; stir; heat for 2 hours.
3. Remove from heat and strain by pouring the mixture through a cheesecloth, squeezing the cloth to release all the liquid.
4. While warm, pour the ointment into glass containers; cool.
5. Apply topically, massaging it until complete absorption, as needed for arthritis pain.

Asthma

If you've ever heard a child with asthma fighting for breath, you'll never forget the wheezing sound or the panic you feel as his or her skin begins to turn blue from lack of oxygen. Asthma is actually a common lung disease that affects people of all ages. In this disease, the trachea and bronchial tubes become inflamed. This causes the airways to narrow, restricting the flow of air, which in turn leads to shortness of breath, difficulty breathing, coughing, wheezing, and a tightness in the chest. An asthma attack can last from a few minutes to a few days and, if severe, can be life threatening.

No cause for the asthma can be determined for many people; however, for others, asthma attacks can be brought on by allergies to molds, pollen, or other allergens, as well as certain foods and drugs. Asthma can also be triggered by cold, damp weather; inhaling dust, smoke, or other irritants; and even infections. Unfortunately, asthma is on the upswing in this country, possibly because of the irritants in our polluted air.

Herbal allies

- Blue Vervain
- coltsfoot
- Echinacea
- Elecampane
- Ginseng
- Goldenseal

- Horehound
- Indian Root
- Passionflower
- Pleurisy root
- Wintergreen
- Yerba sante

QUICK-ACTING ASTHMA TEA

1 teaspoon elecampane root
2 teaspoons horehound herb
1 teaspoon blue vervain leaves
2 cups water

1. Combine the herbs in a pan and cover with water.
2. Bring to a boil; reduce heat and simmer for about 20 minutes; strain and cool.
3. Drink up to two cups a day, a mouthful at a time.

SOOTHING TEA

2 teaspoons powdered Indian root
2 teaspoons granulated echinacea root
2 teaspoons elecampane root
2 cups water

1. Combine the herbs in a pan and cover with the water.
2. Soak for several hours; strain.
3. Take one-half cup two times daily.

Back Pain

Back pain affects most of us at some time in our lives. It can be a dull ache or a sharp burning and stabbing. Sometimes back pain is accompanied by pain that radiates down your leg. This is called sciatica and is a sign that pressure is being placed on the nerves of the spinal cord. Sometimes back pain can be so severe that it limits your activities and renders you bedridden. Often, relaxing the muscles of the back can relieve back pain.

Back pain can have many causes—injury, spasms, sciatica (nerve pain), disc problems, and so on. Long-term resolution requires figuring out what exactly is the root of the problem, but in the meantime these herbs and formulas will relieve pain and release tension, allowing you to move more freely.

Relevant tissue states: tension (spasms), heat (inflammation)
Relevant herbal actions: analgesic, anti-inflammatory, antispasmodic, relaxant

Herbal Allies

- Barberry
- Black Cohosh
- Black Currant
- Black Haw
- Blue Cohosh
- Blue Vervain
- Devil's claw
- Echinacea
- Feverfew
- Ginger
- Goldenrod leaf and flower
- Meadowsweet flower
- Mullein root
- Solomon's seal root
- Wild lettuce

SPINE'S FINE TINCTURE

Makes 4 fluid ounces (40 to 120 doses)

These warming, relaxant, analgesic herbs quell the spasms responsible for most back pain, regardless of whether the pain is acute or chronic, muscular or connective, etc. If you have infused oil made from fresh goldenrod or ginger, use it as a massage oil after you apply this formula topically. For help sleeping, take 1 to 4 drops of tincture of wild lettuce by mouth—this will also contribute more pain-relieving action.

1 fluid ounce tincture of Solomon's seal
1 fluid ounce tincture of ginger
½ fluid ounce tincture of goldenrod
½ fluid ounce tincture of meadowsweet
½ fluid ounce tincture of mullein root (see Tip)
½ fluid ounce tincture of St. John's wort (optional; see Tip)

1. In a small bottle, combine the tinctures. Cap the bottle and label it.
2. Take 1 to 4 drops by mouth 3 to 5 times per day.
3. Additionally, squirt 1 to 4 drops into your palm and rub it into the back muscles.

TIP: If the vertebral discs are impinged or worn away, increase the mullein root to 1 fluid ounce. It specifically supports these tissues. If sciatica or other radiating nerve pain is present, include the tincture of St. John's wort (unless you are taking pharmaceuticals). It regenerates damaged nerve tissue.

WARMING COMPRESS

Makes 1 compress
This simple application provides immediate relief.

16 fluid ounces water
½ cup dried ginger (see Tip)
¼ cup Epsom salts

1. In a small pot with a tight-fitting lid over high heat, combine all the ingredients. Cover and bring to a boil. Reduce the heat and simmer for 5 minutes. Meanwhile, fill a hot water bottle.
2. Soak a cloth in the hot tea, holding it by a dry spot and letting it cool in the air until hot but comfortable to the touch.
3. Lie down and place the wet cloth over your back. Cover with a dry cloth and lay the hot water bottle on top. Get comfortable and let it soak in for 10 to 20 minutes. You should feel warmth, relaxation, and relief from pain.
4. Repeat as often as desired.

TIP: Have pain, but no dried ginger? If all you have on hand is fresh ginger from the grocery store, you can use that, too—sliced, chopped, or grated.

SCIATIC PAIN TEA

2 teaspoons crampbark
2 teaspoons kava kava root
2 cups water

1. Combine the herbs in a pan and cover with water.
2. Bring to a boil; reduce heat; simmer for 30 minutes.
3. Cool and strain.
4. Take up to one cup per day. This tea can help relieve sciatic pain.

ANALGESIC DAILY TEA FOR BACK PAIN

1 teaspoon coltsfoot leaves
2 teaspoons St. John's wort leaves
2 cups boiling water

1. Combine the herbs in a glass container and cover with boiling water; steep for 15 to 30 minutes; strain.
2. Take one-half cup in the morning and one-half cup at night.

SOOTHING BACK PAIN TEA

1 teaspoon chopped valerian root
2 teaspoons white willow bark
2 cups cold water

1. Combine the herbs in a pan and cover with the water.
2. Soak overnight; strain.
3. Take up to one cup a day, a tablespoon at a time.
This tea can help relieve pain caused by nerve irritation.

Bedsores

A bedsore, also called a decubitus ulcer, is an area of damage to the skin that can occur when pressure is applied to an area of the body for a prolonged period of time. The pressure restricts blood flow to the area and also causes irritation, leading to sores.

Skin ulcers are raw, open sores that occur when the top layer of skin cracks and peels away. They are marked by swelling, redness, pain, heat, and inflammation. They may also be infected and full of pus. Bedsores are very common in individuals in casts, as well as those confined to wheelchairs or to bed. In fact, the most common sites for bedsores are the lower back, the buttocks, and the heels. Some authorities estimate that treating bedsores and other decubitus ulcers costs the nation over $1 billion every year.

Herbal remedies

- Burdock
- Echinacea
- Evening primrose
- Marigold
- Nettle
- White Oak

BEDSORE TOPICAL WASH

2 teaspoons marigold flowers
1 teaspoon granulated echinacea root
1 tablespoon white oak bark
2 cups water

1. Combine the herbs in a glass container and cover with the water; soak overnight; strain.
2. Use as a wash periodically throughout the day.

Bites and Stings

Most of us have been bitten or stung by mosquitos, bees, wasps, ants, spiders, ticks, or even more exotic creatures, such as snakes or jellyfishes. We call it a "bite," but most insects and other creatures puncture the skin rather than actually take a bite. It is the substance the animal leaves in the wound and not the wound itself that usually does the damage.

Bites and stings frequently cause localized itching, pain, swelling, and redness. If untreated, any bite or sting can fester and become infected. Even though itching may be severe, resist the urge to scratch, as a secondary infection could result.

Native Americans have had thousands of years to practice using herbs on snakebites. Some of the most helpful herbs for this condition include echinacea and Seneca snakeroot.

Whether it's mosquitoes, black flies, or fire ants, most bug bites are fairly simple: We just need to reduce the inflammation. Bee and wasp stings are a bit more intense: Here, our goals include drawing out the venom, if possible, reducing inflammation, and helping the immune system cope with the venom that has entered the body. Watch for anaphylaxis! If someone stung or bitten is having difficulty breathing, seek help immediately.

Note: If you are stung by a bee or other pest and begin to feel weak, or if you notice any swelling anywhere on the body, call a physician immediately. You may be allergic to the sting and need emergency medical attention. Needless to say, if you are stung by a rattlesnake or other venomous snake, get immediate medical care.

Relevant tissue states: heat (inflammation)
Relevant herbal actions: anti-inflammatory, astringent, lymphatic, immune stimulant

Herbal Allies

- Echinacea
- Seneca snakeroot.
- Black currant
- Ginger
- Ginkgo biloba
- Licorice
- White willow
- Peppermint leaf
- Plantain leaf
- Rose
- Self-heal leaf and flower
- Yarrow leaf and flower

COOLING COMPRESS

Makes 1 compress

Peppermint's menthol provides a cooling sensation to the skin, while at the same time increasing blood circulation and dispersing the irritants from the bite or sting site.

16 fluid ounces water
½ cup dried peppermint leaf

¼ cup Epsom salts

1. In a small pot with a tight-fitting lid over high heat, combine all the ingredients. Cover and bring to a boil. Remove from the heat.
2. Soak a cloth in the hot tea, holding it by a dry spot and letting it cool in the air until hot but comfortable to the touch.
3. Apply the cloth to the bite or sting.

BUG BITE RELIEF SPRAY

Makes 8 fluid ounces (number of applications varies by use)

If you regularly walk through clouds of mosquitoes or black flies or live in an area infested with chiggers, you'll want this cooling, itch-relieving spray stocked for when you come inside.

4 fluid ounces nonalcoholic witch hazel extract or apple cider vinegar
2 fluid ounces tincture of rose
1 fluid ounce tincture of self-heal
1 fluid ounce tincture of yarrow

1. In a bottle with a fine-mist sprayer top, combine all the ingredients. Cap the bottle and label it.
2. Liberally spray wherever you've been bitten.

TOPICAL WASH FOR BITES AND STINGS

2 teaspoons comfrey leaves
2 tablespoons marshmallow leaves
1 tablespoon dried yarrow
1 cup boiling water

1. Combine the herbs in a nonmetallic container and cover with boiling water.
2. Steep for 15 to 30 minutes; strain.
3. Use as a topical wash.

SKIN SOOTHING OINTMENT

1 pound petroleum jelly
4 teaspoons dried agrimony leaves
4 teaspoons dried marigold flowers

1. Melt petroleum jelly in a double boiler.
2. Stir in the herbs and heat for 2 hours until the herbs begin to get crispy.
3. Strain by pouring through cheesecloth.
4. Squeeze the cloth to release all the liquid.
5. While warm, pour the ointment into clean glass containers. Use as needed.

Bronchitis

Bronchitis is an inflammation of the bronchial tubes that can range from a mild case (much like a bad cold) to a severe case, leading to pneumonia. Bronchitis may be accompanied by a fever, severe coughing, thick sputum, difficulty breathing, chills, and a sore throat. Bronchitis usually is caused by an infection but can also occur after inhaling dust, smoke, or other irritants. Repeated bouts of bronchitis can lead to chronic bronchitis, in which the bronchial tubes may become permanently damaged.

When you have a lung infection, don't suppress the cough—it's a vital response! Our goal is to cough when it's productive, so all the irritating or infectious material is expelled as you cough up phlegm, and to reduce the amount of unproductive coughing. If you can't bring up the phlegm, you may find a simple cough developing into pneumonia because of the mucus buildup. (True pneumonia is a serious condition—seek higher care. Meanwhile, take elecampane and garlic—they're your strongest allies for this problem.)

Infection-instigated coughs are usually wet, and the herbs we discuss here assume that's the case. The goal is to get it just a little on the moist side—nice and productive—so you can expel that phlegm.

As with any respiratory condition, an herbal steam is a great remedy all on its own, combating infection and greatly improving blood circulation—which means immune activity—in the lungs. A simple steam with thyme or sage is very good for this problem.

Relevant tissue states: dampness, cold (depressed vitality)
Relevant herbal actions: antimicrobial, astringent, decongestant, diaphoretic, expectorant, pulmonary tonic.

Herbal Allies

- Angelica
- Black Cohosh
- Black Elder
- Canadian fleabane
- Chamomile
- Coltsfoot
- Echinacea
- Elder
- Elecampane root
- Garlic
- Ginger
- Horehound
- Licorice
- Pearly Everlasting Flower
- Peppermint
- Pine
- Queen of the meadow
- Sage leaf
- Seneca snakeroot
- Slippery elm
- Thyme leaf

FIRE CIDER

Makes about 1 quart

Traditional fire cider recipes are blends of pungent and aromatic stimulating expectorants that will heat you up and help you get the gunk out. In this version, we sneak in some immune stimulants and a good source of vitamin C. Do not consume this if you take pharmaceutical blood thinners.

1 whole head garlic, cloves peeled and chopped
1 (2-inch) piece fresh ginger, chopped
¼ cup dried pine needles
¼ cup dried sage leaf
¼ cup dried thyme leaf
¼ cup dried elderberry
¼ cup dried rose hips
2 tablespoons dried elecampane root
2 tablespoons dried angelica root
1 quart apple cider vinegar
Honey or water, for sweetening or diluting (optional)

1.In a quart-size mason jar, combine the garlic, ginger, and remaining herbs.
2.Fill the jar with the vinegar. Cover the jar with a plastic lid, or place a sheet of wax paper under the jar lid before you screw down the ring. (The coating on the bottom of metal mason jar lids corrodes when exposed to vinegar.)
3.Let the herbs macerate in the vinegar for 2 weeks or longer.
4.Strain, bottle, and label the finished fire cider. If the vinegar is too heating to be comfortable on your stomach, add some honey (up to one-fourth the total volume), or dilute your dose with water.
5.Take a shot (about ½ fluid ounce) at the first sign of mucus buildup in the lungs, and every couple hours thereafter until symptoms resolve.

THROAT~SOOTHING TEA

2 teaspoons black cohosh root
2 teaspoons powdered Indian root
2 teaspoons chamomile flower
2 cups water
Honey, to taste

Combine the above herbs in a pan; cover with the water.
Bring to a boil; reduce heat and simmer for 30 minutes; strain.
Add honey if desired. Take one tablespoon in two cups of water several times a day.

SWEET SOOTHING TEA

1 teaspoon marshmallow leaves or flowers

1 teaspoon coltsfoot leaves
1 teaspoon mullein leaves and flowers
½ cup boiling water
Honey

Combine the above herbs; steep one teaspoon of the mixture in the boiling water; strain. Sweeten with honey. Take one-half cup, three or four times a day, hot.

BRONCHITIS TEA #3
1 teaspoon elecampane root
2 tablespoons nettle leaves
1 cup boiling water

Combine the above herbs. Pour the boiling water over the herbs and steep for 30 minutes; strain. Sweeten with honey, if desired. Take up to two cups a day.

BRONCHITIS TEA # 4
1 to 2 slices of fresh ginger root
1 teaspoon pearly everlasting flowers or leaves
1 teaspoon redroot
1 cup boiling water

Combine the above herbs; steep in the boiling water for 30 thirty minutes; strain. Take one-half cup of the tea, three times daily.

Burns and Sunburns

A burn is an injury to the skin or other tissues caused by fire (or another form of heat), electricity, chemicals, or radiation. Burns are classified according to their severity as first-degree, second-degree, or third-degree. In a first-degree burn, the skin will turn red and swell but will not blister. In a few days, there is complete healing, without scarring. The damage from a second-degree burn goes much deeper. The skin turns very red and there is blistering, although the skin heals without scarring. The most severe burn, third-degree, penetrates the skin, destroying both the epidermis and dermis (the segment of the skin beneath the epidermis). A third-degree burn can result in scar tissue formation. Burn tissue can become necrotic and also develop into a serious infection. Skin elasticity can be destroyed. A third-degree burn may actually be less painful than a more superficial first- or second-degree burn because nerve endings in the skin are destroyed. Burns can also occur internally from swallowing very hot liquids or inhaling hot air (such as that from a fire).

A severe burn can cause dangerous systemic damage, such as respiratory tract injury, infection, and shock. Anyone suffering from a severe burn should seek immediate medical attention to counter these potentially life-threatening effects. Herbs, however, can help relieve the pain from a minor burn and encourage rapid healing.

Relevant tissue states: heat
Relevant herbal actions: anti-inflammatory, antimicrobial, antiseptic, vulnerary

Herbal Allies

- Calendula flower
- Coneflower
- Echinacea
- Goldenrod
- Hyssop
- Linden leaf and flower
- Marshmallow
- Peppermint leaf
- Plantain leaf
- Rose petals
- Self-heal leaf and flower
- Sunflower
- Wild Indigo Root

Immediately following a burn, run cold water over the area—the skin retains heat for much longer than you'd expect. (If blisters form in the burned area, be very gentle with them and don't break them before they naturally slough off, if you can avoid it.) Then, gently clean the wound, removing any dirt or contaminant. Apply the herbs, combining antiseptics to prevent infection with cooling, wound-healing herbs to encourage tissue regeneration.

Apply any of the herbal allies in a wash, compress, poultice, or infused honey—don't use oily preparations (like salves) on burns, because they trap the heat in the tissue.

Do not underestimate the power of a marshmallow root poultice! Simply saturate a handful of marshmallow root with enough cold water to make a gloopy mass and apply it to the burn. Cover with gauze and leave in place for 20 minutes. Repeat frequently.

BURN-HEALING HONEY

Makes about 1 pint

Honey is the single best healing agent for burns: If you have nothing but plain honey, you're still in good shape. It gets even better, though, when you infuse these healing herbs into it ahead of time.

½ cup fresh calendula flower
½ cup fresh rose petals
1 pint honey, gently warmed

1.Put the calendula and rose petals in a pint-size mason jar.
2.Fill the jar with the warm honey. Seal the jar and place it in a warm area to infuse for 1 month.
3.In a double boiler, gently warm the closed jar until the honey has a liquid consistency. Strain the infused honey into a new jar, pressing the marc against the strainer to express as much honey as you can.
4.After cooling and cleaning a burn site, apply a layer of the infused honey and cover lightly with a gauze bandage. Refresh the application at least twice a day.

SUNBURN SPRAY

Makes 8 fluid ounces

A few spritzes cool the skin and begin to reduce inflammation.
1 tablespoon dried peppermint leaf
1 tablespoon dried plantain leaf
1 tablespoon dried self-heal leaf and flower
1 tablespoon dried linden leaf and flower
1 quart boiling water
4 fluid ounces rose water

1.Make a hot infusion: In a mason jar, combine the peppermint, plantain, self-heal, and linden. Pour in the boiling water, cover, and steep for 20 minutes.
2.Move the jar to the refrigerator until it's cold.
3.Strain out 4 fluid ounces of the infusion and transfer to an 8-ounce bottle with a fine-mist sprayer top. Use the remaining infusion for compresses or a cooling drink. It will keep, refrigerated, for 3 days.
4.Add the rose water to the spray bottle. Cap the bottle and label it.
5.Apply copiously and frequently. Keep the spray refrigerated when not in use.

BURN POULTICE

1 tablespoon dried coneflower flowers
1 tablespoon dried hyssop flowers

1 tablespoon dried goldenrod flowers
1 tablespoon dried sunflower petals

1. Combine the above ingredients; moisten with boiling water and place between two layers of cheesecloth; let cool and apply to the affected area.
2. When dry, remoisten. Use as often as necessary.

IMMUNITY STRENGTHENER

30 drops echinacea tincture
20 drops wild indigo root tincture
1 cup warm water

1. Combine the above herbs in the warm water.
2. Take up to five times a day.

A burn can weaken the body, leaving you vulnerable to illness and infection. Use this tea to strengthen immunity.

Canker Sores

Canker sores are small sores usually found on the lining of the mouth, although they can also occur on the lips, on the tongue, or in the throat. Also called aphthous ulcers, they can be white or yellow and are surrounded by red, inflamed tissue. These small ulcers can be extremely painful for several days and may be accompanied by fever and swollen lymph glands. Canker sores can be brought on by stress, viral infections, poor dental hygiene, and nutrient deficiencies. Injuries (such as certain dental procedures) can also cause canker sores to develop.

Herbal Allies
- Raspberries
- Black currants
- Big Sagebrush
- Echinacea
- Marigold

ANTI-INFLAMMATORY MOUTHWASH

½ cup barberry tea
½ cup white oak tea
½ cup echinacea tea
½ cup Oregon grape root tea

1. Combine the above ingredients in a glass container with a lid.
2. Use three times a day as a mouthwash. Be sure to swish the liquid around in your mouth for several minutes.

Cold Sores

Cold sores are small, painful, fluid-filled blisters on the mouth caused by the herpes simplex virus. Tingling, itching, and burning may give you a warning that a cold sore is about to erupt. The blisters may appear a few hours or days after the initial warning signs. After a few days, they eventually dry and form a crust. They usually completely heal within a week or two.

Relevant tissue states: heat (inflammation)
Relevant herbal actions: immune stimulant, lymphatic, vulnerary

Herbal Allies

- Burdock
- Echinacea
- Goldenseal
- White Oak
- Yerba Mansa
- Calendula flower
- Chamomile flower
- Linden leaf and flower
- Plantain leaf
- Self-heal leaf and flower
- St. John's wort leaf and flower
- Thyme leaf

COLD SORE COMPRESS

Makes 5 cups dried herb mix (about 50 applications)

This direct application stimulates local immunity and improves tissue quality so your body has the best chance to suppress the virus. For chicken pox or other full-body breakout, take an herb-infused bath with this same formula. Add a bit of baking soda, as it helps with the itching.

1 cup dried calendula flower
1 cup dried plantain leaf
1 cup dried chamomile flower
1 cup dried linden leaf and flower
½ cup dried self-heal leaf and flower
½ cup dried St. John's wort leaf and flower

1. In a large bowl, mix together all the herbs. Store in an airtight container.
2. Make a hot infusion: Prepare a kettle of boiling water. Measure 2 to 3 tablespoons of herbs per quart of water and place in a mason jar or French press. Pour in the boiling water, cover, and steep for 20 minutes. (Meanwhile, fill a hot water bottle.)
3. Soak a cloth in the warm tea, holding it by a dry spot and letting it cool in the air until hot but comfortable to the touch.
4. Lie down and place the wet cloth over the affected area. Cover with a dry cloth and lay the hot water bottle on top. Get comfortable and let it soak in for 10 to 20 minutes.
5. Repeat 2 to 3 times per day.

STEAM VARIATION: You can also perform a steam using these herbs as they're infusing. Simply make a blanket tent, position your face over the steaming pot, and steam yourself with these herbs for a few minutes before you sit with the compress.

COLD SORE BALM

Makes 5 ounces (about a 3-month supply)

This gentle salve is very soothing to irritated cold sores and helps reduce inflammation while making your body's environment less hospitable to the virus.

1 fluid ounce calendula-infused oil
1 fluid ounce plantain-infused oil
½ fluid ounce self-heal–infused oil
½ fluid ounce chamomile-infused oil
½ fluid ounce St. John's wort–infused oil
½ fluid ounce thyme-infused oil
1 ounce beeswax, plus more as needed

1.Make a salve as usual (see here for complete instructions). Make it nice and soft if you'll keep it in little jars; make it slightly firmer if you're using lip balm tubes.
2.Apply liberally to the affected area 3 to 5 times daily.

COLD SORE TEA

1 teaspoon burdock root
1 teaspoon dried and powdered goldenseal root
1 cup boiling water
Honey, to taste

1. Combine the above herbs in a glass container.
2. Pour the boiling water over the herbs; steep for 30 minutes, cool, and strain.
3. You may want to sweeten with honey. Take up to one cup a day.

COLD SORE MOUTHWASH

1 teaspoon echinacea root
1 teaspoon yerba mansa root
1 tablespoon white oak bark
1 cup boiling water

1. Combine the herbs in a glass container.
2. Pour the boiling water over the herbs.

3. Steep 30 minutes, cool, and strain. Use the solution as a wash to treat cold sores.

Constipation

Formerly called "costiveness," constipation refers to any irregularity in, or absence of, bowel movements. The frequency of bowel movements depends on your diet, your physical makeup, and your physical habits. Most people have one movement a day, but some people may go two days or more and not suffer from constipation. However, the longer waste products remain in the colon, the more water will be absorbed, and the drier and more compact the waste will become.

Constipation can occur because of a poor diet, inadequate water intake, nervous tension, insufficient exercise, drug use, poor or inconsistent toilet habits, and laxative overuse. A number of diseases, including thyroid problems, circulatory disorders, and colon disturbances (such as fistulas, inflammation, polyps, obstructions, and tumors) can also cause constipation.

Relevant tissue states: cold (stagnation), dryness, tension
Relevant herbal actions: bitter, carminative, demulcent, hepatic, laxative

Herbal Allies

- Angelica
- Barberry
- Boneset
- Cascara Sagrada
- Cayenne
- Chicory
- Dandelion root
- Ginger
- Marshmallow
- Milk thistle seed
- Oregon Grape
- St. John's wort leaf and flower
- Sunflower

Sometimes, constipation is simply a sign of dehydration—drink some water! If it's a chronic issue, it may be an indication of a food allergy or simply a sign that you're not getting sufficient fiber in your diet. A good, thick, cold infusion of marshmallow solves both problems: It rehydrates better than water alone, and it includes a lot of polysaccharides and fibers that help move stool along.

Constipation, especially when ongoing, can be traced back to sluggish liver function. Bile produced by the liver is a digestive fluid, but it also lubricates the intestines; when production is low, things can get stuck. Bitters and carminatives help spur digestive function, and liver-restorative herbs (hepatics) such as milk thistle can reestablish normal function.

BOWEL-HYDRATING INFUSION

Makes 2½ cups dried herb mix (enough for 14 to 18 quarts of tea)

A bit tastier than solo marshmallow, this is a great solution for the type of constipation that often afflicts people with dry constitutions. If you have hard-to-pass, dry, little "rabbit pellet" bowel movements, this is for you. Drink a quart or more every day.

1 cup dried linden leaf and flower

1 cup dried marshmallow root
¼ cup dried cinnamon bark
¼ cup dried licorice root

1.In a medium bowl, mix together all the herbs. Store in an airtight container.
2.Make a cold infusion: Measure 2 to 4 tablespoons of herbs per quart of water and place in a mason jar or French press. Pour in cold or room-temperature water and steep for 4 to 8 hours before straining.

BOWEL~MOTIVATING TINCTURE

Makes 4 fluid ounces (30 to 60 doses)

These bitters and carminatives will spur the bowels to movement by stimulating bile flow and intestinal peristalsis.

1½ fluid ounces tincture of dandelion root
1½ fluid ounces tincture of St. John's wort
½ fluid ounce tincture of angelica root
½ fluid ounce tincture of ginger

1.In a small bottle, combine the tinctures. Cap the bottle and label it.
2.Take 2 to 4 drops every 20 minutes until relief occurs.

BOWEL~SOOTHING TEA

One large handful of boneset flowers
One large handful of dandelion flowers
4 ounces cascara bark
2 quarts water
Honey

Combine the above herbs in a pan and cover with two quarts of water; bring to a boil; boil until the mixture reduces to one quart; strain.
Take one cup before breakfast and one at bedtime. You may want to add honey to sweeten.

PURIFYING DIGESTIVE TEA

2 teaspoons cascara sagrada
3 to 4 slices ginger root
1 teaspoon cayenne

1 teaspoon Oregon grape root
2 cups boiling water

Combine the above herbs in a pan and cover with two cups of boiling water; steep for 30 to 45 minutes, cool, and strain. Take one tablespoon at a time, up to two cups per day.

Cough and Cold

The common cold is an upper respiratory tract infection caused by one of more than 100 viruses. Symptoms of a common cold include watery eyes, runny or stuffy nose (rhinitis), head congestion (with a mild, moderate, or severe headache), fatigue, sneezing, and coughing. The cough that often accompanies a cold is the body's attempt to clear the air passage of mucus, dust, or other substances that cause irritation. Your sense of taste and smell may be decreased, and you may run a fever or suffer from chills. A general aching feeling of discomfort and listlessness (malaise) may be present. There may be a sore throat, ranging from mild to severe, as the cold develops. Any or all of these symptoms may be present.

Relevant tissue states: heat (irritation) or cold (depressed vitality), dryness or dampness
Relevant herbal actions: antitussive, astringent, decongestant, demulcent, diaphoretic, expectorant, pulmonary tonic

Herbal Allies

- Agrimony
- Black currant
- Black Elder
- Blue Vervain
- Boneset
- Chamomile
- Coltsfoot
- Echinacea
- Elecampane
- Fennel seed
- Ginger
- Gingko Biloba
- Goldenrod
- Goldenseal
- Horehound
- Indian Root
- Licorice
- Mullein
- Osha
- Oxeye Daisy
- Peppermint
- Pine
- Pleurisy Root
- Queen of the Meadow
- Speedwell
- White cedar leaf tips
- Wild Cherry
- Wild Indigo
- Yarrow
- Yerba mansa
- Yerba sante
- Marshmallow
- Mullein leaf
- Sage leaf
- Thyme leaf

For herbs to work best, we need to differentiate between a hot, dry, irritated cough and one that is wet, but cold and unproductive. When the lungs are dry, you'll have a racking, relentless cough; we use moistening herbs to correct this. Wet lungs rattle or gurgle and are most likely a response to infection. See Bronchitis/Chest Cold/Pneumonia or Cold and Flu.

LUNG~LUBRICATING TEA

Makes 2¾ cups dried herb mix (enough for 18 to 22 quarts of tea)

For dry, hot lungs, these soothing and moistening herbs bring relief from a racking, unrelenting cough.

1 cup dried marshmallow root
1 cup dried mullein leaf
½ cup fennel seed
¼ cup dried licorice root, or to taste
Honey, for extra soothing (optional)

1. In a medium bowl, mix together all the herbs. Store in an airtight container.
2. Make a cold infusion: Measure 2 to 4 tablespoons of herbs per quart of water and place in a mason jar or French press. Pour in cold or room-temperature water and steep for 4 to 8 hours.
3. Strain the liquid and drink directly, or warm, if desired.
4. Add honey (if using) for extra soothing.

ANTITUSSIVE OXYMEL

Makes about 1 quart (20 to 60 doses)

An oxymel is simply a blend of vinegar and honey, which combines the astringent and stimulating effects of the vinegar with the moistening and soothing aspects of the honey. Adding lung-specific herbs makes this a go-to for coughs of all kinds.

⅓ cup dried pine needles
⅓ cup dried sage leaf
⅓ cup dried thyme leaf
¼ cup dried ginger
1 quart apple cider vinegar
Honey, as needed for topping off the jar

1. In a quart-size mason jar, combine the herbs.
2. Fill the jar four-fifths full with vinegar; top off with honey.
3. Cover the jar and let macerate for 4 weeks.
4. Strain and bottle the oxymel. Cap the bottle and label it.
5. Take 1 to 3 tablespoons as needed.

COUGH SYRUP

2 teaspoons coltsfoot leaves
1 tablespoon wild plum root
2 teaspoons mullein leaves
2 cups boiling water
1 pound honey

1. Combine the above herbs in the boiling water; in a nonmetallic container steep for 30 minutes and strain.
2. Add one pound of honey, heating and stirring until the honey is dissolved; cool and store in a glass container.
3. Take one tablespoon at a time, as needed.

SOOTHING COUGH AND COLD FORMULA

30 drops echinacea tincture
20 drops wild indigo root tincture
2 cups white cedar leaf tips tea

1. Combine the above ingredients and take half a cup at a time, hot.
2. Take up to three times a day.

LAKOTA COUGH AND COLD FORMULA

1 teaspoon goldenseal root
1 teaspoon mullein leaves
1 teaspoon osha root
1 teaspoon pleurisy root
1 teaspoon yerba mansa root
2 teaspoons yerba sante leaves
2 cups boiling water

1. Combine the above herbs and cover with the boiling water; steep for 30 minutes, cool, and strain.
2. Take two tablespoons at a time, as needed, up to two cups a day.

LUMBEE COUGH AND COLD FORMULA

3 teaspoons goldenrod leaves

4 teaspoons horehound leaves
2 teaspoons white pine inner bark
4 cups boiling water

1. Combine the above herbs in a cheesecloth; tie closed with a string.
2. Place the bag in the boiling water; boil for 15 minutes; cool; remove the bundle.
3. Take half a cup of the hot mixture at a time, as needed, up to two cups a day.

QUICK-ACTING COUGH AND COLD FORMULA

4 teaspoons agrimony leaves
2 teaspoons mullein leaves
2 teaspoons blue vervain leaves
1 teaspoon oxeye daisy
3 teaspoons horehound leaves
2 teaspoons speedwell
2 cups boiling water

1. Combine the above herbs in a nonmetallic container and cover with the boiling water; steep for 30 minutes, cool, and strain.
2. Take a tablespoonful every three hours, as needed, up to two cups a day.

EXPECTORATING COUGH AND COLD TEA

2 teaspoons boneset herb
2 teaspoons licorice root
2 to 3 slices ginger root
2 teaspoons wild cherry bark
2 cups boiling water

Combine the above herbs in a nonmetallic container and cover with the boiling water; steep for 30 minutes, cool, and strain. Take one to two tablespoons at a time, up to two cups a day, as needed, for a dry tickling cough.

DECONGESTANT TEA

2 slices fresh ginger
2 teaspoons pleurisy root
1 cup boiling water

1. Combine the herbs in a glass container; pour one cup of boiling water over the herbs; steep for 30 minutes, cool, and strain.
2. Take a tablespoon at a time, up to two cups a day. This tea is good for bronchial congestion.

ANTITUSSIVE FLOWER TEA

1 teaspoon elderflowers
1 teaspoon yarrow flowers
1 cup boiling water

1. Combine the herbs in a nonmetallic container and cover with one cup of boiling water; steep for 20 minutes and strain.
2. Drink hot every two hours, as needed.

QUICK-ACTING MULLEIN COUGH SYRUP

1 cup of mullein tea
1 pound honey

1. Combine the above ingredients in a pan and heat until the honey is liquid.
2. Remove from heat, cool, and pour into a glass container. Take a tablespoon at a time, as needed.

ELECAMPANE COUGH SYRUP

2 cups of elecampane tea
1 pound honey

1. Combine the tea with the honey and heat on low. Stir to dissolve the honey; when dissolved, remove the mixture from the heat.
2. When cool, pour into glass containers and seal.
3. Take two tablespoons at a time, as needed, up to one cup a day.

HOREHOUND LOZENGES

1½ cups horehound leaves
1½ cups water

3 cups sugar
3 tablespoons corn syrup

1. Place the horehound leaves in a pan and cover with the water.
2. Bring the mixture to a boil and boil for 20 minutes.
3. Remove from the heat and cool. Strain the solution and add the sugar and corn syrup.
4. Place back on the heat, bring to a boil, then reduce heat to medium.
5. Cook until the mixture reaches 300°F (hard-crack stage).
6. Pour the syrup onto a large buttered baking sheet; cool, then break into one-inch pieces.
7. Use as you would any cough drop.

Cramps

Cramping muscles are involuntary muscle contractions. They can be very painful and tight. Muscle cramps can be caused by cold temperatures, dehydration, overexercise, nutrient imbalances, and restricted blood flow to the muscles. Muscle cramps also can be caused by an imbalance in the body's electrolytes (electrolytes in the body include calcium, magnesium, potassium, and sodium). Muscle cramps usually occur in the legs, where they can often be severe enough to keep you from walking. Muscle cramps can also occur in the arms, the back, and in virtually any and every muscle of the body.

Relevant tissue states: heat (inflammation), tension
Relevant herbal actions: anodyne, nervous tropho-restorative, relaxant, rubefacient

Herbal Allies

- Black Cohosh
- Ginseng
- Wintergreen
- Yerba Mansa
- Cinnamon bark
- Ginger
- Goldenrod leaf and flower
- Meadowsweet flower
- Peppermint essential oil
- Wild lettuce
- Yarrow leaf and flower

A bit of delayed-onset muscle soreness after a hard day's work or an intense workout is normal. Rest well! Recovery time is when muscles grow stronger; if you don't give them time to recover fully, you'll confound your efforts. Eat well, too: providing the necessary nutrients speeds recovery. Bone broth with seaweed added is a great place to start.

MUSCLE-WARMING OINTMENT

20 drops yerba mansa tincture
4 ounces wintergreen oil
1 pound petroleum jelly

1. Thoroughly mix the above herbs with the petroleum jelly.
2. Use as an ointment to relieve muscle cramps.

MUSCLE CRAMP TEA

2 teaspoons black cohosh root
1 tablespoon ginseng root
2 cups water

1. Combine the above herbs in a pan and cover with two cups of water; bring to a boil; reduce heat and simmer for 30 minutes, cool, and strain.
2. Take two to three tablespoons up to six times a day.

MUSCLE RUB

Makes 8 fluid ounces (100+ applications, 30-day supply)

These warming herbs increase local circulation, simultaneously reducing inflammation and soothing tension. If, after applications, you're still in a lot of pain when it's time to go to bed, take 1 to 2 drops of wild lettuce tincture for further relief.

2 fluid ounces ginger-infused oil
2 fluid ounces goldenrod-infused oil
2 fluid ounces tincture of ginger
2 fluid ounces tincture of meadowsweet
80 drops peppermint essential oil or cinnamon essential oil (or both!)

1.In a small bottle, combine the infused oils, tinctures, and essential oil(s). Cap the bottle and label it, including Shake well before each use.
2.Hold your palm over the bottle's mouth and tilt to deposit a small amount in your palm. Rub between your hands to warm the treatment, and apply to the painful joints.
3.Massage the liniment into the joints until your hands no longer feel oily. Really work the liniment into the tissue.
4.Repeat the application 3 to 5 times per day. More is better!

DIARRHEA

Diarrhea is marked by frequent and excessive discharge of watery fecal material. Diarrhea can occur because of bacterial or viral infections or intestinal parasites. Certain chemicals and drugs can cause diarrhea, as can certain diseases, such as ulcerative colitis and cancer. Emotional stress can also bring on diarrhea. Food allergies, drinking caffeine or alcohol, or eating unripe fruit or spoiled food can also bring on an attack.
Excessive or prolonged diarrhea can cause dehydration, which can interfere with the absorption of nutrients. Diarrhea can be especially dangerous in children because they cannot tolerate much fluid loss.

Relevant tissue states: laxity (barrier compromise), dampness
Relevant herbal actions: astringent, demulcent

Herbal Allies
- Agrimony
- Alumroot
- Angelica
- Barberry
- Blackberry
- Black Currant

- Canadian fleabane
- Catnip
- Cayenne
- Cinnamon bark
- Ginger Root
- Marshmallow
- Meadowsweet flower
- Mint
- Pine Bark
- Plantain leaf
- Raspberry
- Rose
- Self-heal leaf and flower
- Strawberry leaf
- Witch hazel
- Yarrow
- Yellow Dock

When the lining of the bowels loses integrity, excess fluid is lost. To counteract this directly, astringent herbs restore healthy tone to the mucous membranes, so water stays in the body where it belongs. Once this is accomplished, it's a good idea to follow up with some soothing demulcent herbs—especially if the diarrhea has been going on for a while, as that causes dehydration, which must be corrected.

ASTRINGENT TEA

Makes 2¼ cups dried herb mix (enough for 14 to 18 quarts of tea)

The tannins in these herbs help bind lax tissues back together so fluids stay where they belong and barriers keep their integrity. Drink a quart of tea over the course of the day.

1½ cups dried self-heal leaf and flower
½ cup dried meadowsweet flower
¼ cup rose petals

1. In a medium bowl, mix together all the herbs. Store in an airtight container.
2. Make a hot infusion: Prepare a kettle of boiling water.
3. Measure 2 to 3 tablespoons of herbs per quart of water and place in a mason jar or French press.
4. Pour in the boiling water, cover, and steep for 20 minutes or until cool enough to drink.

TINCTURE VARIATION: If you prefer, make a tincture blend using the same proportions: Combine 1½ fluid ounces tincture of self-heal, ½ fluid ounce tincture of meadowsweet, and ¼ fluid ounce tincture of rose petal. Take 1 to 6 drops every 20 minutes until relief occurs.

CINNAMON POWDER CAPSULES

Makes 20 to 24 capsules

When cinnamon is extracted into water—as an infusion or decoction—its demulcent quality is emphasized. However, if you swallow a capsule of the powder, the capsule dissolves in your GI tract and releases the dry powder, which then absorbs excess water and exerts an astringent effect on the intestinal lining. This quells diarrhea quite nicely. The Capsule Machine, a handy manual capsule-filling device, helps with this recipe quite a lot.

20 to 24 empty gelatin capsules, size "00"
2 tablespoons powdered cinnamon

1. Fill the capsules with the cinnamon powder.
2. Take 1 to 3 capsules when you have diarrhea. If relief isn't obtained within an hour, take another dose.

QUICK AND EASY DIARRHEA TEA

3 tablespoons agrimony leaves
2 tablespoons self-heal
4 cups water

1. Combine the herbs in a pan; cover with the water; bring to a boil; reduce heat and simmer for 30 minutes; cool and strain.
2. Drink as needed, up to one cup a day.

SOOTHING DIARRHEA TEA

2 teaspoons alumroot
2 teaspoons blackberry leaves
2 teaspoons angelica seeds
1 teaspoon Oregon grape root
2 cups boiling water

1. Combine the above herbs in a nonmetallic container.
2. Pour the boiling water over the herbs and steep for 30 minutes; strain; take as needed, up to one cup a day.

IROQUOIS TEA

2 teaspoons raspberry leaves
2 teaspoons strawberry leaves

2 tablespoons yarrow
2 teaspoons yellow dock root
2 cups boiling water

1. Combine the herbs in a glass container; pour the boiling water over the herbs; steep for 30 minutes; cool and strain.
2. Take up to one cup a day. The Iroquois made a similar tea to treat bloody diarrhea.

Fatigue

Fatigue is more than just being tired. Instead, fatigue is a prolonged or excessive decrease in the ability to function, over and above what normal exertion would cause. Those who push themselves to the point of physical exhaustion are certainly familiar with fatigue. However, fatigue can be a symptom of more than overexertion; it is a symptom of a number of conditions including anemia, circulatory problems (such as angina pectoris, atherosclerosis, and high blood pressure), chronic fatigue syndrome, diabetes, hepatitis, inflammatory bowel disease, multiple sclerosis, and respiratory conditions including pneumonia and pleurisy.

Relevant tissue states: cold (depletion, depression, exhaustion)
Relevant herbal actions: adaptogen, exhilarant, stimulant

Herbal Allies

- Angelica
- Ashwagandha root
- Blackberry
- Gingko Biloba
- Ginseng
- Gotu Kola
- Licorice root
- Mirabilis
- Pulsatilla
- Raspberry
- St. John's Wort
- Strawberry leaf
- Tulsi leaf

Fatigue is an indication that something is impairing recovery. Most of the time, it's simply a lack of sleep. (Believe it or not, healthy adults need 8 to 10 hours of sleep a night—every night—and most Americans only get 6 on weekdays, 8 on weekends!) Even if your fatigue is not immediately relieved by a good night's sleep, it's still important to prioritize sleep. While there can be other factors in play (malnutrition, chronic illness, stress, pharmaceutical side effects, etc.), sleep is irreplaceable.

To counter fatigue, we should not underestimate the importance of movement for building energy. A little bit of motion can grow into greater kinetic energy if you cultivate it, gently and consistently. Tai chi and qigong are excellent for this.

While you're working on that, we'll draw on the talents of our adaptogens and uplifting, stimulating herbs to help break through the fog and push forward.

SHAKE-IT-OFF FORMULA

Makes 3 fluid ounces (45 to 90 doses)

1 fluid ounce tincture of licorice
1 fluid ounce tincture of ashwagandha
1 fluid ounce tincture of tulsi

1.In a small bottle, combine the tinctures. Cap the bottle and label it.

2.Take 1 to 2 drops, at morning and noontime. Feel free to take additional doses whenever you need a boost.

UP~AND~ABOUT MORSELS

Makes about 24 pieces

These tasty, restorative treats are a good way to get a substantial dose of beneficial herbs. This format is particularly useful because it provides the full complement of plant compounds instead of just those that are water soluble or alcohol soluble, as happens with a tea or tincture.

¼ cup powdered ashwagandha root
¼ cup powdered tulsi leaf
¼ cup powdered milk thistle seed
¼ cup powdered nettle leaf
3 tablespoons powdered licorice root
¾ cup nut butter
½ cup honey

Unsweetened shredded coconut, cocoa powder, powdered cinnamon, powdered ginger, cayenne, or whatever seems tasty to you, for coating

1.In a large bowl, blend the powders together.
2.Add the nut butter and honey. Stir to form a thick "dough."
3.Roll the dough into balls about the size of a walnut (1 inch).
4.Roll the balls in your coating of choice.
5.Eat 1 to 4 per day.

PICK~ME~UP TEA

1 teaspoon Ginkgo biloba leaves
1 teaspoon dried mirabilis root
1 teaspoon dried ginseng root
1 teaspoon pulsatilla herb
1 teaspoon gotu kola leaves
1 teaspoon St. John's wort leaves
4 cups boiling water

1. Combine the above herbs in a glass container; cover with the boiling water; steep for 30 minutes; strain.
2. Take as needed.

INVIGORATING TEA

1 teaspoon blackberry leaves
1 teaspoon strawberry leaves
1 teaspoon raspberry leaves
2 cups boiling water
Honey

1. Combine the above herbs in a glass container; cover with the boiling water; steep for 10 minutes; strain.
2. Sweeten with honey if desired. Drink as needed.

Fever

"Normal" body temperature is generally considered to be 98.6°F, although that number may vary between individuals, or even in the same individual at different times of the day. For example, our body temperature is lowest in the early morning and highest in the late afternoon. However, a fever is considered to be any temperature above 100°F. A fever is usually a sign that the body is fighting off some type of infection.

Whether or not to treat a fever is a very controversial subject. In my opinion, fever is the body's way of repairing itself and should not be suppressed. However, fever in children and in adults with heart illness and other disorders is sometimes serious and may need to be treated.

Relevant tissue states: heat, dryness (dehydration)
Relevant herbal actions: diaphoretic, refrigerant

Herbal Allies

- Angelica
- Boneset
- Cayenne
- Catnip leaf and flower
- Elderflower
- Garlic
- Ginger
- Juniper
- Marigold
- Osha Root
- Oxeye Daisy
- Peppermint leaf
- Sage leaf
- Skullcap
- Thyme leaf
- Tulsi leaf
- Wild Indigo Root
- Wild lettuce
- Yarrow leaf and flower

Fever is your friend: It's a vitally important immune response—and herbalists aren't the only ones saying so! The American Academy of Pediatrics released a clinical report in 2011 that stated: "It should be emphasized that fever is not an illness but is, in fact, a physiologic mechanism that has beneficial effects in fighting infection." So, don't give in to fever phobia—help your body do its work.

Stay hydrated! Almost all serious problems associated with fever come not from the fever itself but from runaway dehydration. If a person is too nauseous to keep down fluids, sitting in a warm bath is a good way to rehydrate.

Finally, remember that temperatures are relative to individuals. Children run hot, elders run cool, and constitution influences your baseline body temperature. A limp and unresponsive person at 99°F is in more trouble than an active, alert person at 101°F. So, always look at the person more closely than the thermometer.

FEVER~INDUCING TEA

Makes 3 cups dried herb mix (enough for 18 to 24 quarts of tea)

Often we want to help fever come on strong, with the help of our stimulating diaphoretics. These will help a fever be more productive, and they can also help the fever be more bearable because they cause the body to sweat. Drink a big mug of this tea whenever a fever is low and lingering and you want to boost it into an effective heat.

1 cup dried tulsi leaf
½ cup dried sage leaf
½ cup dried thyme leaf
½ cup dried yarrow leaf and flower
¼ cup dried angelica root
¼ cup dried ginger
1 garlic clove, sliced, for a real kick (optional)

1. In a medium bowl, mix together all the herbs. Store in an airtight container.
2. Make a hot infusion: Prepare a kettle of boiling water. Measure 2 to 3 tablespoons of herbs per quart of water and place in a mason jar or French press. Add the garlic (if using). Pour in the boiling water, cover, and steep for 20 minutes.
For best effect, reheat before drinking and drink very hot.

FEVER~BREAKING TEA

Makes 1¾ cups dried herb mix (enough for 14 to 24 pints of tea)

If the fever is too hot to tolerate, these relaxing diaphoretics and refrigerants will relieve tension and release the heat without stimulating more fire. The wild lettuce in the mix will make you sleepy, which is good—sleep is your best healing mechanism. Go to bed!

½ cup dried catnip leaf and flower
½ cup dried elderflower
½ cup dried peppermint leaf
¼ cup dried wild lettuce leaf and stalk
1 pint boiling water

1.In a medium bowl, mix together all the herbs. Store in an airtight container.
2.Make a hot infusion: Measure 1 to 2 tablespoons of herbs and place in a pint-size mason jar. Pour in the boiling water, cover, and steep for 20 minutes or until cool. Drink this tea slightly cooler than usual.
3.Sip on a mugful when you want to reduce a fever.

FEVER RELIEF TEA

1 teaspoon angelica root
1 teaspoon ground ivy leaves
1 teaspoon barberry berries
2 teaspoons peppermint leaves
2 teaspoons blue vervain leaves
1 tablespoon dried yarrow
1 teaspoon catnip leaves
1 cup boiling water

1. Combine the above herbs.
2. Place one tablespoon of the mixture in a cup; pour the boiling water over the herbs; steep for 30 minutes; strain.
3. Take up to one cup a day.

QUICK-ACTING FEVER TEA

1 teaspoon echinacea root
1 teaspoon white willow root
1 cup water

1. Combine the roots in a pan and cover with the water.
2. Bring to a boil; reduce heat and simmer for 30 minutes; cool and strain.
3. Take half a cup, up to four times a day.

Food Intolerances

Food sensitivities are extremely common and run the gamut from mild to life-threateningly severe. They cause all manner of gastrointestinal upsets—heartburn, IBS, bloating, and more—but can also contribute to systemic inflammation, neurological problems, and autoimmunity. In our opinion, everyone should periodically assess for sensitivity to a few common foods: Gluten, dairy, soy, corn, eggs, and nightshades (potatoes, tomatoes, peppers, eggplant, etc.) are all common culprits. A 30-day elimination period similar to what's described on Whole30.com, during which you avoid the suspect food entirely and track the severity of your symptoms, is the best way to identify if you have a sensitivity to a particular food.

Once your individual trigger foods are identified and eliminated from your diet, there's still some cleanup and reset work to do—that's where herbs really shine. A cup or two of herb-infused broth and a quart of gut-healing infusion in a day will have you feeling like a new person in no time.

Relevant tissue states: heat (inflammation), laxity (barrier compromise)
Relevant herbal actions: bitter, carminative, demulcent, hepatic, nervine, nutritive, relaxant, vulnerary

Herbal Allies

- Angelica
- Barberry
- Bayberry
- Blue Cohosh
- Calendula flower
- Catnip leaf and flower
- Chamomile flower
- Coneflower
- Dandelion
- Echinacea
- Fennel seed
- Ginger
- Kelp
- Licorice root
- Marshmallow
- Meadowsweet flower
- Oregon grape
- Peppermint
- Plantain leaf
- Self-heal leaf and flower
- St. John's wort leaf and flower
- Tulsi leaf
- Yarrow leaf and flower

Flatulence, or gas, is often a symptom of indigestion and can develop when we eat too fast or too much. It can also occur because of allergies or enzyme deficiencies and is a sign that our bodies are not breaking down the foods that we eat. For example, those people whose bodies do not make the enzyme lactase can't adequately digest the sugars in dairy products. The milk sugars in these products then ferment in the colon, causing gas. High-fiber foods can also cause flatulence, as can beans and cabbage.

Indigestion refers to any gastrointestinal disturbance, such as an upset stomach. Indigestion can occur if you eat too fast, eat too much, eat while emotionally upset, or, for some people, eat the wrong foods. Caffeine, high-fiber foods, alcohol, and carbonated drinks are often indigestion culprits. Sometimes allergies can cause indigestion. Indigestion can be a symptom of a number of diseases, including pancreatitis, ulcers, gastritis, and cholecystis. Often, however, there is no known cause for indigestion.

GUT-HEAL TEA

Makes 4⅓ cups dried herb mix (enough for 20 to 40 quarts of tea)

This blend of digestive herbs combines all the actions needed to restore healthy function to the stomach, intestines, and liver. It is the single most-frequently recommended formula in our practice and is open to a wide degree of individual customization: If you have lots of gut cramping, add more chamomile and fennel. If you're constitutionally dry, add more marshmallow. If you run very hot, omit the ginger. If there's an herb you don't like, just leave it out, and if there's one you particularly love, add more! Drink a quart or more every day.

½ cup dried calendula flower
½ cup dried plantain leaf
½ cup dried chamomile flower
½ cup dried tulsi leaf
⅓ cup dried catnip leaf and flower
⅓ cup fennel seed
⅓ cup dried peppermint leaf
⅓ cup dried marshmallow leaf
¼ cup dried ginger
¼ cup dried licorice root
¼ cup dried yarrow leaf and flower
¼ cup dried St. John's wort leaf and flower (see Tip)

1. In a large bowl, mix together all the herbs. Store in an airtight container.
2. Make a hot infusion: Prepare a kettle of boiling water. Measure 2 to 3 tablespoons of herbs per quart of water and place in a mason jar or French press. Pour in the boiling water, cover, and steep for 20 minutes or until cool enough to drink.
TIP: Omit the St. John's wort if you are concurrently taking pharmaceuticals.

BUILD-UP BROTH

Makes about 3 quarts

Bone broth is very healing to the gut, especially when the bones have bits of collagen (gristle) attached. The amino acids in these parts help restore intestinal integrity, which is compromised by the food allergy reaction. Adding herbs enhances these healing and anti-inflammatory activities. If you feel particularly awful, forego solid food for a day and just have lots of broth! One more reason to get in the bone broth habit: Broth made from bones with collagenous tissue still attached is rich in glucosamine and chondroitin. These nutrients are utilized by the body to rebuild healthy joints and connective tissues. You can buy glucosamine and chondroitin as supplements, but bone broth is a cheaper source and has so many other additional benefits!

1 cup dried calendula flower

¼ cup dried dandelion root
¼ cup fennel seed
¼ cup dried ginger
¼ cup dried kelp
Bones (such as from 1 rotisserie chicken; 6 pork chop bones; 1 lamb or beef shank; or the bones, head, and tail from 2 medium fish—really, any bones will do . . .)
3 quarts water, plus more as needed
1 tablespoon apple cider vinegar
Oyster, shiitake, or maitake mushrooms, for their nutritive and healing properties (optional)
Salt
Freshly ground black pepper

1. In a large pot over high heat, combine the herbs, bones, water, vinegar, and mushrooms (if using). Season with salt and pepper. Bring to a boil. Sustain boiling for 4 to 8 hours. Check often and add enough water to replace what has boiled away.
2. Strain the liquid and reserve. Compost the bones and herb marc, if desired.
3. Drink a mug of warm broth 2 to 3 times per day.

STOP-FLATULENCE TEA

1 teaspoon dried angelica root
2 teaspoons peppermint leaves
1 teaspoon bee balm leaves
1 cup boiling water

1. Combine the herbs in a container.
2. Take one tablespoon of the herb mixture and cover with the boiling water; steep for 20 to 30 minutes; strain. Take as needed.

COLON-SOOTHING TEA

2 teaspoons bee balm leaves
2 teaspoons peppermint leaves
2 teaspoons chamomile flowers
1 cup boiling water

1. Combine the herbs in a container.
2. Take one tablespoon of the mixture and cover with the boiling water; steep for 30 minutes; strain. Take as needed.

QUICK-ACTING FLATULENCE TEA

1 teaspoon catnip leaves
1 teaspoon grated ginger root
2 teaspoons dandelion leaves
2 cups boiling water

1. Combine the herbs and cover with the boiling water; steep for 20 to 30 minutes; strain.
2. Take as needed.

GUT-CLEARING TEA

1 teaspoon blue cohosh root
1 teaspoon coneflower root
1 cup boiling water

1. Combine the above herbs in a glass container.
2. Pour the boiling water over the herbs; steep for 30 minutes; cool and strain. Take as needed, up to one cup a day.

DAILY DIGESTIVE TEA

1 teaspoon angelica root
1 teaspoon grated ginger root
2 teaspoons chamomile flowers
2 teaspoons peppermint leaves
1 cup boiling water

1. Combine the above ingredients in a container.
2. Take one tablespoon of the herb mixture and place in the boiling water; steep for 30 minutes; cool and strain. Take as needed, up to two cups a day.

PEPPERY INDIGESTION TEA

1 teaspoon licorice root
1 teaspoon peppermint leaves
2 cups boiling water

1. Combine the above herbs in a nonmetallic container and cover with the boiling water; steep for 15 to 20 minutes; strain.
2. Take as needed, up to one cup a day.

Hangover

Everyone knows what a hangover is, even if they have never experienced one firsthand. Excessive alcohol intake dehydrates the body, which is why those suffering from a hangover have a dry mouth and are thirsty. Too much alcohol can also elevate and then drastically drop blood sugar levels, leading to headache, irritability, shakiness or dizziness, and fatigue. Alcohol depletes the body of certain nutrients and can cause fat to build up in the liver. It also causes the stomach to excrete too much acid, which can lead to heartburn, nausea, and vomiting. No wonder a hangover feels so awful.

Relevant tissue states: heat (inflammation), dryness (dehydration), laxity (barrier compromise)
Relevant herbal actions: anodyne, antiemetic, anti-inflammatory, relaxant

Herbal Allies

- Barberry
- Bayberry
- Betony leaf and flower
- Catnip
- Chaparral
- Chamomile flower
- Ginger
- Goldenseal
- Linden leaf and flower
- Licorice root
- Marshmallow
- Milk thistle seed
- Oregon Grape
- Plantain leaf
- Peppermint
- Self-heal leaf and flower
- St. John's wort leaf and flower

The number-one hangover preventive and simplest remedy is milk thistle capsules. Milk thistle is one of the few herbs that are very effective in capsule form, and almost all commercially available brands are good quality. The best strategy is to take 2 capsules with a big glass of water before you start drinking, another 2 before bed, and 2 more in the morning. Sometimes this will prevent you from getting a hangover at all!

TAKE-IT-EASY NEXT DAY INFUSION

Makes about 3¼ cups dried herb mix (enough for 20 to 28 quarts of tea)
This gentle tea calms the most common hangover symptoms and helps with rehydration to boot. Best to mix it up before the big party, so it'll be ready when you need it. Drink a quart or more, slowly, over the course of the day.

½ cup dried betony leaf and flower
½ cup dried plantain leaf
½ cup dried calendula flower
½ cup dried chamomile flower
⅓ cup dried linden leaf and flower

⅓ cup dried marshmallow leaf
⅓ cup dried self-heal leaf and flower
1 tablespoon dried licorice root
1 tablespoon dried ginger
¼ cup dried St. John's wort leaf and flower

1.In a medium bowl, mix together all the herbs. Store in an airtight container.
2.Make a hot infusion: Prepare a kettle of boiling water. Measure 2 to 3 tablespoons of herbs per quart of water and place in a mason jar or French press. Pour in the boiling water, cover, and steep for 20 minutes or until cool enough to drink.

TIP: Omit the St. John's wort if you are concurrently taking pharmaceuticals.

NO~FUSS HANGOVER TEA

1 teaspoon ripe barberry berries
1 teaspoon Oregon grape root
2 cups boiling water

1. Combine the herbs in a nonmetallic container and cover with the boiling water; steep for 30 minutes; cool and strain.
2. Take up to one cup a day, diluted in plenty of cool water.

QUICK~ACTING HANGOVER TEA

1 teaspoon bayberry root
1 teaspoon dried goldenseal root
1 teaspoon Oregon grape root
2 cups boiling water

1. Combine the herbs in a nonmetallic container and cover with the boiling water; steep for 30 minutes; strain.
2. Place a tablespoon of the mixture in an 8-ounce glass of water.
3. Drink several glasses throughout the day.

SPICY HANGOVER TEA

1 teaspoon catnip leaves
1 teaspoon peppermint leaves

1 teaspoon dried chaparral leaves
2 cups boiling water

1. Combine the herbs in a nonmetallic container and cover with the boiling water; steep for 20 to 30 minutes; strain.
2. Drink half a cup at a time, up to two cups a day.

Headache

Headaches are very common and can be dull and steady, stabbing, gnawing, or throbbing. There are many kinds of headaches with many different causes. Sometimes tension, fatigue, or stress can cause a headache. Problems with the eyes, ears, nose, throat, or teeth can bring on a headache, as can allergies, injuries, infection, tumors, and any number of diseases. Headaches are also big business. In fact, Americans spend in excess of $1 billion each year buying medicines to help combat headaches. Most people take nonsteroidal anti-inflammatory drugs (NSAIDs) such as aspirin, ibuprofen, or indomethacin, or even stronger painkillers. But these drugs have unwanted, and sometimes serious, side effects, including ulcers and an increased tendency to bleeding. Herbs can offer a safer alternative.

Relevant tissue states: heat or cold, damp or dry, tense or lax
Relevant herbal actions: anodyne, anti-inflammatory, astringent, circulatory stimulant, relaxant

Herbal Allies

- Betony leaf and flower
- Catnip
- Chamomile flower
- Feverfew
- Peppermint
- Pleurisy root
- White Willow
- Wintergreen
- Ginger
- Linden leaf and flower
- Marshmallow
- Meadowsweet flower
- Sage leaf
- Tulsi leaf
- Wild lettuce

Headaches arise from a variety of imbalances. Some are simple one-off causes—dehydration, sleep debt, dietary excesses, alcohol, caffeine, medications. For those, you want quick pain relief while you supply what's missing or simply wait for the body to recover. (When unsure of where to start, turn to betony.)

For long-term relief, it's important to identify your individual triggers, as well as the underlying patterns that contribute to your pain; this takes some experimentation. The following herbal remedies are designed to address the most common types of headaches we see, but try different combinations of herbs to refine the remedy and make it as personal as possible. If you have recurrent headaches and find this helps, drink a quart or more every day as a preventive.

COOLING HEADACHE TEA

Makes 3¼ cups dried herb mix (enough for 22 to 28 quarts of tea)

If a headache makes you turn red-faced, and the pain feels hot, sharp, and very sensitive to the touch, this is for you. This kind of headache often results from tension, stress or anxiety, sinus congestion, or direct nerve pain. These herbs cool, relax (be aware the wild lettuce may make you sleepy), and drain.

1 cup dried betony leaf and flower
1 cup dried meadowsweet flower
½ cup dried linden leaf and flower
½ cup dried marshmallow leaf
¼ cup dried wild lettuce leaf and stalk

1.In a medium bowl, mix together all the herbs. Store in an airtight container.
2.Make a hot infusion: Prepare a kettle of boiling water. Measure 2 to 3 tablespoons of herbs per quart of water and place in a mason jar or French press. Pour in the boiling water, cover, and steep for 30 to 40 minutes. Drink warm or cool. One cup of this tea should begin to give some relief.

WARMING HEADACHE TEA

Makes 3¼ cups dried herb mix (enough for 22 to 28 quarts of tea)

If, when your headaches strike, you have a pale face and the pain feels cold, dull, and broad, try this blend. This type of headache is often caused by hypothyroidism, liver congestion, and circulatory stagnation. These herbs warm, gently astringe, and improve circulation. (If caffeine usually works as a headache remedy for you, try this.) If you have recurrent headaches and find this helps, drink a quart or more every day as a preventive.

1 cup dried betony leaf and flower
1 cup dried tulsi leaf
½ cup dried chamomile flower
½ cup dried sage leaf
¼ cup dried ginger

1.In a medium bowl, mix together all the herbs. Store in an airtight container.
2.Make a hot infusion: Prepare a kettle of boiling water. Measure 2 to 3 tablespoons of herbs per quart of water and place in a mason jar or French press. Pour in the boiling water, cover, and steep for 30 to 40 minutes. Drink warm to hot. One cup of this tea should begin to give some relief.

PEPPERY HEADACHE TEA

1 teaspoon feverfew leaves
1 teaspoon peppermint leaves

1 cup boiling water
Honey

1. Combine the above herbs in a nonmetallic container and cover with the boiling water; steep for 30 minutes; strain.
2. Add honey to taste. Take a tablespoon at a time, up to one cup a day.

SOOTHING HEADACHE TEA

1 teaspoon catnip leaves
2 teaspoons feverfew leaves
1 to 2 cups boiling water

1. Combine the catnip and the feverfew in a glass container.
2. Pour one to two cups of boiling water over the herbs; steep for 30 minutes; strain.
3. Take up to one cup a day, a tablespoon at a time.

HEARTBURN/REFLUX/GERD

Heartburn is burning stomach pain that can spread up into your throat. Heartburn occurs when hydrochloric acid from your stomach backs up into the esophagus. This condition can result if you gulp your food or drink too much caffeine or alcohol. It can also occur if you eat while stressed or eat certain foods (such as spicy or fatty foods). Antacids are commonly taken for heartburn, but herbs can be just as effective.

Note: If you suffer from heartburn, avoid peppermint. Although it is helpful in treating indigestion and other stomach problems, it can relax the esophageal sphincter and actually increase the tendency toward heartburn.

Relevant tissue states: heat (inflammation), laxity
Relevant herbal actions: bitter, carminative, demulcent, vulnerary

Herbal Allies

- Barberry
- Bayberry
- Catnip leaf and flower
- Chamomile flower
- Chaparral
- Coriander
- Dandelion root
- Fennel seed
- Ginger

- Hops
- Kelp
- Licorice root
- Linden leaf and flower
- Marshmallow
- Meadowsweet flower
- Oregon grape
- Self-heal leaf and flower
- St. John's wort leaf and flower
- Yellow Dock

Contrary to what you might expect, heartburn is most often caused by low levels of stomach acid. When stomach acid is low, it causes a chain of problems in the digestive system that ultimately increase upward-moving pressure in the abdomen. This weakens the "trapdoor" between the stomach and the esophagus—when that's compromised, acid is more likely to splash up through and irritate the unprotected tissue there.

Reducing stomach acid production (with antacids or acid-blocking pharmaceuticals) temporarily relieves pain, but makes the underlying problem worse. To address heartburn, first we have to heal existing damage in the esophagus or stomach (inflammation and ulcers). Then we can work to restore normal acid levels to prevent recurrence.

That stomach-esophagus "trapdoor" (the lower esophageal sphincter, LES) can also be compromised by poor alignment and stress. When in a state of stress, saliva production decreases and digestive movement is inhibited. A rest-and-digest state of mind is required to retain the proper resting tone of the LES. This starts by being present with your food—slow down, chew thoroughly, take your time.

MARSHMALLOW INFUSION

Makes 1 quart

If you have active heartburn, the first thing you need is a good cold infusion of marshmallow root. Keep this on hand for when there's an attack and to heal the damaged tissue in the esophagus. When heartburn happens, just sip on this slowly and you'll feel relief in no time.

2 to 4 tablespoons dried marshmallow root

In a quart-size mason jar, combine the marshmallow with enough cold or room-temperature water to fill the jar. Cover and steep for 4 to 8 hours. Keep refrigerated, where each batch will last for 2 to 3 days.

PREVENTIVE BITTER TINCTURE

Makes 3½ fluid ounces (30 to 60 doses)

To restore normal stomach acid levels and reduce the conditions for heartburn to develop, take these drops before every meal.

1 fluid ounce tincture of dandelion root
½ fluid ounce tincture of catnip
½ fluid ounce tincture of chamomile
⅓ fluid ounce tincture of fennel
⅓ fluid ounce tincture of meadowsweet
⅓ fluid ounce tincture of self-heal
½ fluid ounce tincture of St. John's wort (see Tip)

1. In a small bottle, combine the tinctures. Cap the bottle and label it.
2. Take ½ to 1 dropperful 10 minutes before eating.

TIP: Omit the St. John's wort if you are concurrently taking pharmaceuticals.

QUICK~ACTING HEARTBURN TEA

1 teaspoon dried angelica root
1 teaspoon crushed juniper berries
1 cup boiling water

1. Combine the herbs in a nonmetallic container and cover with the boiling water; steep for 20 to 30 minutes; strain.
2. Take a tablespoon at a time, as needed.

SOOTHING HEARTBURN TEA

1 teaspoon catnip leaves
1 teaspoon oxeye daisy herb
1 cup boiling water

1. Combine the herbs in a non-metallic container and cover with the boiling water; steep for 30 minutes; strain.
2. Take a tablespoon at a time, as needed.

Hypertension

The list of circulatory disorders is almost endless and includes heart disease, strokes, hypertension, and atherosclerosis, to name a few. These and other circulatory conditions are the number-one cause of death in this country, killing nearly one million Americans every year.

As we age, our body's ability to keep a proper equilibrium between blood clotting and blood liquefaction begins to go awry. On the one hand, blood must clot if we are to keep from bleeding to death, yet, on the other hand, it must be free flowing and liquid in order to travel easily through the body's blood vessels. The older we get, the "stickier" our blood gets, and our blood's ability to flow diminishes. When this occurs, the stage is set for blood clots, clogged arteries, strokes, and heart attacks.

Relevant tissue states: heat, tension
Relevant herbal actions: hypotensive, nervine, relaxant, sedative

Herbal Allies

- Black Cohosh
- Black Currant
- Burdock
- Cayenne
- Dandelion
- Garlic
- Ginger
- Gingko Biloba
- Ginseng
- Goldenseal
- Gotu Kola
- Kelp
- Linden leaf and flower
- Marshmallow
- Raspberry
- Rose
- Slippery Elm
- Yarrow leaf and flower

Occasional high blood pressure is normal—it's a part of the natural response to stressful situations. Over time, though, high blood pressure can cause or worsen other cardiovascular problems. Herbs offer a nice suite of actions to reduce high blood pressure, often by addressing root causes rather than merely acting symptomatically.

It's worth noting that high blood pressure isn't always bad: New information indicates that hypertension that develops in the elder years may actually help reduce the risk of dementia.

SOFTHEARTED TEA

Makes 2 cups dried herb mix (enough for 12 to 16 quarts of tea)

Reducing stress makes a big difference, so herbs that can relax the mind while soothing the physical heart are ideal. For those with very dry constitutions, prepare this as a cold infusion instead. Drink a quart or more every day.

1 cup dried linden leaf and flower

½ cup dried marshmallow leaf
½ cup dried rose petals

1.In a small bowl, mix together all the herbs. Store in an airtight container.
2.Make a hot infusion: Prepare a kettle of boiling water. Measure 2 to 3 tablespoons of herbs per quart of water and place in a mason jar or French press. Pour in the boiling water, cover, and steep for 20 minutes or until cool enough to drink.

FREE-FLOWING CIRCULATION TEA

1 teaspoon burdock root
1 teaspoon goldenseal root
1 teaspoon cayenne
2 teaspoons slippery elm bark
2 slices ginger root
3 cups boiling water

1. Combine the above herbs in a nonmetallic container, and pour the boiling water over them. Steep for 30 minutes, cool, and strain.
2. Take up to one cup a day, two tablespoons at a time.

ANTI-CONGESTIVE TEA

2 teaspoons black cohosh root
4 teaspoons ginkgo biloba leaves
2 cups boiling water

1. Combine the above herbs in a nonmetallic container, and pour the boiling water over them. Soak for 30 minutes, cool, and strain.
2. Take two to three tablespoons at a time, up to six times a day.

ARTERIOSCLEROSIS PREVENTIVE TEA

2 to 3 ginger slices
2 teaspoons Ginkgo biloba leaves
1 teaspoon ginseng leaves
2 cups boiling water

1. Combine the herbs in a nonmetallic container and cover with the boiling water.

2. Steep for 30 minutes, cool, and strain.
3. Take up to half a cup per day.

Indigestion/Dyspepsia

Indigestion refers to any gastrointestinal disturbance, such as an upset stomach. Indigestion can occur if you eat too fast, eat too much, eat while emotionally upset, or, for some people, eat the wrong foods. Caffeine, high-fiber foods, alcohol, and carbonated drinks are often indigestion culprits. Sometimes allergies can cause indigestion. Indigestion can be a symptom of a number of diseases, including pancreatitis, ulcers, gastritis, and cholecystis. Often, however, there is no known cause for indigestion.

Relevant tissue states: cold (stagnation), tension
Relevant herbal actions: bitter, carminative, relaxant

Herbal Allies

- Angelica
- Barberry
- Bayberry
- Blue Cohosh
- Catnip leaf and flower
- Chamomile flower
- Coneflower
- Dandelion root
- Echinacea
- Fennel seed
- Ginger
- Licorice root
- Oregon Grape
- Peppermint leaf
- Sage leaf

If you're having chronic digestive discomforts, take a hard look at your diet to see if you have any food sensitivities. Lucky for you, though, indigestion is a problem for which herbal quick fixes are ready at hand—read on for two simple, portable solutions.

PRE-EMPTIVE BITTER TINCTURE

Makes 4 fluid ounces (60 to 120 doses)

Indigestion often means just that—incomplete digestion. This formula stimulates all your digestive fluids—saliva, stomach acid, bile, and pancreatic enzymes—so digestion is as thorough and complete as possible.

1 fluid ounce tincture of dandelion root
1 fluid ounce tincture of sage
1 fluid ounce tincture of catnip
1 fluid ounce tincture of chamomile

1. In a small bottle, combine the tinctures. Cap the bottle and label it.
2. Take 1 to 2 drops 10 minutes before eating.

CARMINATIVE TINCTURE

Makes 4 fluid ounces (60 to 120 doses)

This formula warms the body's core, stimulating your digestive organs and keeping the bowels from getting sluggish. If peppermint isn't your style, substitute angelica.

1½ fluid ounces tincture of ginger
1 fluid ounce tincture of fennel
1 fluid ounce tincture of peppermint (see headnote)
½ fluid ounce tincture of licorice

1. In a small bottle, combine the tinctures. Cap the bottle and label it.
2. Take 1 to 2 drops after each meal, or whenever your guts feel uncomfortably stuck.

DIGESTIVE TEA

1 teaspoon blue cohosh root
1 teaspoon coneflower root
1 cup boiling water

1. Combine the above herbs in a glass container.
2. Pour the boiling water over the herbs; steep for 30 minutes; cool and strain.
3. Take as needed, up to one cup a day.

STRONG DIGESTIVE TEA

1 teaspoon angelica root
1 teaspoon grated ginger root
2 teaspoons chamomile flowers
2 teaspoons peppermint leaves
1 cup boiling water

1. Combine the above ingredients in a container.
2. Take one tablespoon of the herb mixture and place in the boiling water; steep for 30 minutes; cool and strain.
3. Take as needed, up to two cups a day.

QUICK-ACTING DIGESTIVE TEA

1 teaspoon licorice root
1 teaspoon peppermint leaves
2 cups boiling water

1. Combine the above herbs in a nonmetallic container and cover with the boiling water; steep for 15 to 20 minutes; strain.
2. Take as needed, up to one cup a day.

Insomnia

Insomnia is any difficulty in sleeping. Some people find it difficult to fall asleep, while others can fall asleep easily but don't stay asleep. Nearly one-fourth of all Americans have an occasional problem sleeping, but some people (as much as 10 percent of the American population) suffer from chronic insomnia. Insomnia can occur for a number of reasons, including stress and nervous tension, excessive intake of caffeinated drinks, and irregular sleeping habits.

Insomnia can lead to fatigue and an inability to function at an optimal energy level during the day. Irritability, daytime drowsiness, and memory impairment often affect those suffering from insomnia.

Relevant tissue states: heat (agitation), tension
Relevant herbal actions: hypnotic, relaxant, sedative

Herbal Allies

- Ashwagandha root
- Betony leaf and flower
- Catnip leaf and flower
- Chamomile flower
- Hops
- Linden leaf and flower
- Passionflower
- Rose
- Valerian
- Wild lettuce

Wild animals don't have insomnia. Hikers in the wilds don't either, actually. According to a 2013 study in the journal Current Biology, just a few days in an outdoor environment, with no artificial light exposure, is enough to reestablish normal circadian rhythms—even in people who are habitual "night owls" in their city lives. This tracks with a large and growing body of evidence that indicates that our electrically lit environments are directly responsible for most sleep disturbances we experience.

Reducing evening exposure to bright lights—including TV, computer, and smartphone screens—is one of the most important steps you can take to fight insomnia. Dimming lights and avoiding screens for at least an hour before bed, and taking the herbal remedies offered here, are sure ways to improve both the quantity and quality of your sleep.

END~OF~THE~DAY ELIXIR

Makes 4 fluid ounces (60 to 120 doses)

This blend of relaxants and gentle sedatives doesn't force sleep but helps relieve the tension, anxiety, and distraction that make it difficult to transition into sleep. This formula (and any herbs taken to aid in sleep) is best taken in "pulse doses," which is much more effective than taking the total dose all at once right at bedtime. It gives the herbs time to start working in your system and emphasizes to the body that it's time to transition into sleep.

1 fluid ounce tincture of chamomile

1 fluid ounce tincture of betony
¾ fluid ounce tincture of ashwagandha
½ fluid ounce tincture of catnip
½ fluid ounce tincture of linden
¼ fluid ounce honey (plain or rose petal–infused)

1.In a small bottle, combine the tinctures and honey. Cap the bottle and label it.
2.One hour before bedtime, take 1 to 2 drops.
3.Thirty minutes before bedtime, take another 1 to 2 drops.
4.At bedtime, take the final 1 to 2 drops.

SLEEP! FORMULA

Makes 4 fluid ounces (60 to 120 doses)

For this formula, we recruit wild lettuce, the strongest hypnotic (sleep-inducing) herb in this book. This is especially helpful if part of what's keeping you up at night is physical pain, as wild lettuce also has a pain-relieving effect. This formula, like End-of-the-Day Elixir, is best taken in "pulse doses."

2 fluid ounces tincture of wild lettuce
1 fluid ounce tincture of betony
½ fluid ounce tincture of chamomile
½ fluid ounce tincture of linden

1.In a small bottle, combine the tinctures. Cap the bottle and label it.
2.One hour before bedtime, take 1 to 2 drops.
3.Thirty minutes before bedtime, take another 1 to 2 drops.
4.At bedtime, take the final 1 to 2 drops.

INSOMNIA RELIEF TEA

1 teaspoon chamomile flowers
1 teaspoon hops
1 teaspoon valerian root
1 cup boiling water

1. Combine the above herbs.
2. Take one tablespoon of the mixture and cover with the boiling water; let steep for 30 minutes; strain.
3. Drink warm, as needed, half a cup at a time.

SWEET DREAMS TEA

2 teaspoons catnip leaves
1 teaspoon hops
2 teaspoons chamomile flower
2 teaspoons passionflower
1 cup boiling water

1. Combine the above herbs in a glass container; cover with the boiling water; steep for 30 minutes; cool and strain.
2. Take one hour before bedtime.

Menstrual cycle irregularities

The irregularities include various disruptions of the menstrual cycle. Each is addressed slightly differently, but a few overarching actions emerge that help with all of them: nourishing the body, improving circulation, and stimulating the liver and kidneys to clear away used-up hormones.

Delayed or absent menses may be due to a lack of adequate nourishment, especially protein, or to disruptions in hormone levels. (Sometimes these share a cause. A high-sugar diet is nutrient-poor, and the havoc it wreaks on blood sugar levels has a cascade effect that disrupts hormone balance. Stress makes us tend to eat gratifying but poor-quality food, and excessive stress-response hormones interfere with the normal actions of estrogen and progesterone.)

Irregular cycles, with no predictable pattern, may also be due to poor nourishment, liver stagnation or strain, or an irregular lifestyle—especially erratic sleep habits. The daily cycle shapes the monthly cycle, like small and large gears interlocking in a watch.

Overheavy bleeding generally comes from hormones not clearing efficiently at the liver, though it may also be connected with the development of fibroids or polyps. If heavy bleeding persists, seek medical attention.

Finally, let's talk about the most common menstrual ailment: dysmenorrhea, or menstrual pain, which usually begins just before menstruation, may occur in the lower abdomen or the lower back (and sometimes even into the thighs). Other accompanying symptoms may include nausea, vomiting, headache, and either constipation or diarrhea. This condition affects more than half of all women.

There are two types of dysmenorrhea, primary and secondary. In primary dysmenorrhea, there is no underlying pain causing the disorder. It is thought that the pain occurs when uterine contractions reduce blood supply to the uterus. This may occur if the uterus is in the wrong position, if the cervical opening is narrow, and due to lack of exercise.

Secondary dysmenorrhea is when the pain is caused by some gynecological disorder, such as endometriosis (when the endometrium, the tissue that lines the uterus, abnormally grows on surfaces of other structures in the abdominal cavity), adenomyosis (in-growth of the endometrium into the uterine musculature), lesions, inflammation of the fallopian tubes, or uterine fibroids. Uterine fibroids are tumors of the uterus that are not usually cancerous. Also known as myomas, these masses occur in nearly one-quarter of all women by the age of forty. Some women with uterine fibroids may have no symptoms. However, if symptoms are present they include increased frequency of urination, a bloated feeling, pressure, pain, and abnormal bleeding.

Relevant tissue states: cold (stagnation), laxity
Relevant herbal actions: astringent, carminative, circulatory stimulant, emmenagogue, nutritive, rubefacient

Herbal Allies

- Angelica
- Ashwagandha root
- Betony leaf and flower
- Black Cohosh
- Blue Vervain
- Chamomile flower
- Crampbark
- Dandelion leaf
- Elecampane
- Feverfew
- Ginger
- Goldenrod leaf and flower
- Kelp
- Marigold
- Milk thistle seed
- Nettle leaf
- Passionflower
- Peppermint
- Pulsatilla
- Raspberry
- Sage leaf
- Self-heal leaf and flower
- St. John's Wort
- Tulsi leaf

STEADY CYCLE TEA

Makes 3½ cups dried herb mix (enough for 20 to 28 quarts of tea)

These herbs provide substantial nourishment and a bit of gentle kidney, lymphatic, and endocrine stimulation. Long-term use of a formula like this has been the major factor in improvement for a great many of our clients with menstrual irregularities of all types. Add ginger if you run cold, betony if you're frequently anxious, and peppermint for taste (if you like it). Drink a quart or more every day.

1 cup dried nettle leaf
1 cup dried dandelion leaf
½ cup dried goldenrod leaf and flower
½ cup dried self-heal leaf and flower
¼ cup dried tulsi leaf
¼ cup dried kelp

1. In a small bowl, mix together all the herbs. Store in an airtight container.
2. Make a long infusion: Prepare a kettle of boiling water. Measure 2 to 3 tablespoons of herbs per quart of water and place in a mason jar or French press. Pour in the boiling water, cover, and steep for 8 hours or overnight.

BLEED ON! TEA

Makes 3 cups dried herb mix (enough for 20 to 26 quarts of tea)

To bring on menstruation, drink this tea for 3 days to 1 week prior to the expected start of your next period. Drink this tea very hot for best results. Reheat as necessary and drink a quart or more over the course of the day. For a stronger effect, take a drop of angelica tincture together with each cup of tea.

1 cup dried chamomile flower
1 cup dried tulsi leaf
⅓ cup dried goldenrod leaf and flower
⅓ cup dried ginger
⅓ cup dried angelica root

1. In a small bowl, mix together all the herbs. Store in an airtight container.
2. Make a hot infusion: Prepare a kettle of boiling water. Measure 2 to 3 tablespoons of herbs per quart of water and place in a mason jar or French press. Pour in the boiling water, cover, and steep for 20 minutes or until cool enough to drink.

DAILY SOOTHING MENSTRUAL TEA

2 teaspoons black haw root or bark
2 teaspoons passionflower
2 cups cold water

1. Combine the above herbs in a pan and cover with the cold water; soak overnight; strain.
2. Take half a cup, up to four times daily.

DYSMENORRHEA TEA

2 teaspoons black cohosh root
1 teaspoon crampbark
1 teaspoon black haw root or bark
1 teaspoon pulsatilla
2 cups water

1. Combine the above herbs in a pan and cover with the water; bring to a boil and boil for 10 minutes; cool and strain.
2. Take half a cup, up to four times a day.

CRAMP RELIEF TEA

1 teaspoon St. John's wort leaves
1 teaspoon raspberry leaves
1 cup boiling water

1. Combine the herbs in a glass container and cover with the boiling water; steep for 15 minutes; strain.
2. Drink as needed to relieve cramps.

Nausea and Vomiting

Nausea is an unpleasant feeling that you are about to vomit. It is often accompanied by excess salivation and sometimes stomach cramping. A number of diseases and conditions can cause nausea, including food poisoning (and other bacterial infections), viral infections, overeating or overdrinking, gallstones, pancreatitis, and cancer. It can also occur because of motion sickness, headache, or pregnancy. Sometimes unpleasant smells or tastes, and even emotional anxiety, can bring on nausea.

Relevant tissue states: heat (agitation), tension (spasm)
Relevant herbal actions: antiemetic, carminative, relaxant

Herbal Allies

- Bayberry
- Bee Balm
- Catnip leaf and flower
- Chamomile flower
- Chaparral
- Fennel seed
- Ginger
- Horehound
- Oregon Grape
- Peppermint leaf
- Yerba mansa

One way or another, nausea almost always comes from food—a sensitivity, some indigestion, various potential infections. Especially if nausea happens frequently, look closely at your diet—keeping a journal can be helpful—to identify any patterns that occur around its appearance. Maybe when you eat on the run, or eat wheat products, or have really fiery spices—whatever it is for you, the only way to identify it is to pay attention in an organized way.

After a bout of vomiting, some warm, slightly weak Calming Tea can be the easiest thing to drink for quite some time. Then slowly reintroduce broth, then soup, then stew . . . gradually progressing from food prepared to be very warm and moist to food that is more cool and dry, like salad.

Both of the following formulas are also excellent for morning sickness. If you feel you can't get anything down at all, just one drop of ginger tincture all by itself on the tongue can be helpful, or even just smelling strong ginger tea.

CALMING TEA

Makes 3¼ cups dried herb mix (enough for 20 to 26 quarts of tea)

For most cases of nausea, this combination of the best herbal antiemetics should help very quickly. If you know you prefer (or dislike) the flavor of one of these ingredients, feel free to adjust its proportion. This also helps as a preventive—if prone to nausea, drink a quart or more every day.

1 cup dried catnip leaf and flower
1 cup dried chamomile flower
½ cup dried peppermint leaf
½ cup fennel seed
¼ cup dried ginger

1. In a medium bowl, mix together all the herbs. Store in an airtight container.
2. Make a hot infusion: Prepare a kettle of boiling water. Measure 2 to 3 tablespoons of herbs per quart of water and place in a mason jar or French press. Pour in the boiling water, cover, and steep for 20 minutes or until cool enough to drink.
3. Drink a cupful, slowly, in small sips. If the nausea is very severe, just sit for a while and inhale the scent rising off the hot tea.

GINGER EMERGENCY FORMULA

Makes 5 fluid ounces (60 to 120 doses)

This mixture of tinctures is one to keep in your herbal first aid kit at all times. You never know when nausea will strike, and a quick herbal relief will be very welcome. Make this with ginger-infused honey if you have the time to prepare that in advance.

2 fluid ounces tincture of ginger
1 fluid ounce tincture of catnip
1 fluid ounce tincture of chamomile
1 fluid ounce honey

1. In a small bottle, combine all the ingredients. Cap the bottle and label it.
2. Take 1 to 2 droppersful every 20 minutes until relief occurs.

ANTIEMETIC TEA

1 teaspoon grated ginger root
1 teaspoon yerba mansa root
1 teaspoon peppermint leaves
2 cups boiling water

1. Combine the above herbs in a nonmetallic container and cover with the boiling water; steep for 30 minutes; cool and strain.
2. Take as needed, a tablespoon at a time, up to two cups a day.

NAUSEA-SOOTHING TEA

1 teaspoon catnip leaves
1 teaspoon chamomile flowers
1 cup boiling water

1. Combine the above ingredients in a nonmetallic container and cover with the boiling water; steep for 20 to 30 minutes; cool and strain.
2. Take as needed.

Rash

A skin rash is a temporary eruption on the skin that usually looks like small red or pink bumps. It may or may not itch. There may be scaly, round, or oval patches on the skin. A rash is usually a symptom of some other condition and can indicate a disease such as measles or chickenpox, an insect bite, an allergic reaction, a nutritional deficiency, or even dry skin.

Relevant tissue states: heat (inflammation), dryness or dampness, laxity
Relevant herbal actions: anti-inflammatory, astringent, demulcent

Herbal Allies

- Burdock
- Calendula flower
- Comfrey
- Echinacea
- Evening Primrose
- Goldenseal
- Kelp
- Licorice root
- Marshmallow
- Oregon grape
- Plantain leaf
- Rose
- Self-heal leaf and flower
- Slippery Elm
- St. John's wort leaf and flower
- Strawberry
- Uva-ursi leaf
- White oak
- Yarrow leaf and flower
- Yellow Dock

A sudden appearance of a rash generally means you've come into contact with some kind of irritant—an irritating plant, a toxic chemical, or perhaps an insect bite or sting. Wash the area well with soap and water. Then apply insights from basic herbal energetics: If the rash is dry, use moistening herbs and preparations; if it's damp and oozy, use drying agents.
If there doesn't seem to have been any contact with an irritating plant, chemical, or other direct trigger, the rash may be an external reflection of an internal imbalance. Allergies can cause this, of course, as well as overworked internal detoxification systems.

DRY RASH SALVE

Makes 9 ounces (60-day supply)

Salves are emollient due to their oil and wax content, especially when they have a moisturizing oil, like olive oil, as the base. In this simple formula, the herbs' healing and anti-inflammatory effects enhance the emollient effect.

3 fluid ounces calendula-infused oil
3 fluid ounces plantain-infused oil
2 fluid ounces licorice-infused oil
1 ounce beeswax, plus more as needed

1.Prepare a salve as usual (see here for complete instructions).
2.Gently apply a thin layer to the affected area at least twice a day.

WEEPY RASH POULTICE

Makes 4½ cups dried herb mix (enough for 12 to 18 poultices)

Contact with poison ivy and similar plants often produces a rash with fluid-filled blisters. These call for astringents, and those are best delivered in a water extract—a poultice or compress.
Learn to identify the plants that cause contact rash in your area! Poison ivy, poison oak, and poison sumac all grow in the US. Check out poison-ivy.org for great pictures and details about how to make a positive identification, as well as how to tell them apart from benign look-alike plants.

1 cup dried calendula flower
1 cup dried rose petals
1 cup dried self-heal leaf and flower
½ cup dried St. John's wort leaf and flower
½ cup dried uva-ursi leaf
½ cup dried yarrow leaf and flower
Boiling water, to make the poultice

1.In a large bowl, mix together all the herbs. Store in an airtight container.
2.Measure 4 to 6 tablespoons of the herb mixture and place in a heat-proof dish.
3.Pour just enough boiling water over the herbs to get them fully saturated—not so much that they're swimming. Let the herbs soak for 5 minutes.
4.Apply the mass of herbs, warm and wet, to the affected area. Cover with a cloth. Keep in place for 5 to 10 minutes, then gently pat dry.
5.Repeat 1 to 3 times per day.

TIP: If you don't have these herbs on hand, plain green or black tea bags will do the trick! Just get them warm and wet, apply them over the rash, and let them sit in place for 20 minutes.

SKIN-SOOTHING TEA

1 teaspoon burdock root
1 teaspoon Oregon grape root
1 teaspoon echinacea root
1 teaspoon yellow dock root
2 cups water

1. Combine the above herbs in a pan and cover with the water. Bring to a boil; reduce heat and simmer for 10 to 15 minutes; cool and strain.

2. Take a tablespoon at a time, up to half a cup a day.

RASH WASH

1 teaspoon comfrey root
1 teaspoon white oak leaves or bark
1 teaspoon slippery elm bark
2 cups water

1. Place the herbs in a container and cover with the water; bring to a boil and boil for 20 to 30 minutes; cool and strain.
2. Use as a topical wash, as needed.

Sinusitis/Stuffy Nose

Sinusitis is an inflammation of the sinuses, marked by sinus congestion, headache, and pain around the eyes or cheeks. There may be a nasal discharge, fatigue, cough, fever, earache, and an increased susceptibility to nasal infections.

Sinusitis can be caused by allergies, bacterial or fungal infections, and viral infections (such as the common cold). However, nasal injury, a deviated septum (the separator between the two nasal passages), a swollen conchae (the spiral air warmers in the nose), nasal polyps, or narrow sinuses can also cause sinusitis, as can cigarette smoke, dusty or dry air, or even infected tonsils or teeth.

Relevant tissue states: heat (inflammation), laxity (mucous membranes)
Relevant herbal actions: antifungal, anti-inflammatory, antimicrobial, astringent, decongestant, demulcent

Herbal Allies

- Bayberry
- Black Elder
- Calendula flower
- Echinacea
- Garlic
- Ginger
- Gingko Biloba
- Ginseng
- Goldenrod leaf and flower
- Goldenseal
- Licorice
- Pau D'Arco
- Pine
- Rose
- Slippery Elm
- Valerian
- White Willow
- Wild Indigo
- Witch Hazel
- Marshmallow
- Sage leaf
- Thyme leaf
- Uva-ursi leaf
- Yerba mansa

Runny nose is a vital response to a cold or the flu! Believe it or not, mucus is full of antibodies. Drying it up with pharmaceutical decongestants makes the tissue more susceptible to infection. Keeping mucous membranes at a happy medium—not too dry, not too drippy—helps shorten the illness and prevent complications.

If not connected to a full respiratory infection, or if chronic or recurrent, the cause of symptoms is likely a complex of bacterial, fungal, and viral components. (This is why it can persist even after multiple rounds of antibiotics.) Antimicrobial herbs are less specific than antibiotic drugs, which is a benefit in this case, meaning that they can counteract a variety of pathogens and compromised states simultaneously.

Grating fresh horseradish and breathing its fumes, or eating prepared horseradish or wasabi, is a great way to clear the sinuses. If you've been blowing your nose a lot and the skin is irritated, some soft, simple salve or lanolin is very soothing.

SINUS-CLEARING STEAM BATH

Makes 2 cups dried herb mix (enough for 4 to 8 steams)

Steaming is a universal treatment across cultures for any respiratory system troubles, including those related to the sinuses. The combination of hot steam and the evaporating volatile oils from the herbs makes it very difficult for pathogens to survive and stimulates immune response in the mucous membranes.

1 cup dried pine needles
½ cup dried sage leaf
½ cup dried thyme leaf
½ gallon water
5 garlic cloves, chopped, per steam (optional)

1. In a small bowl, mix the pine, sage, and thyme. Store in an airtight container.
2. Make and execute an herbal steam: In a medium pot over high heat, boil the water.
3. Place the pot on a heat-proof surface, someplace where you can sit near it, and make a tent with a blanket or towel.
4. Add ¼ to ½ cup of the herb mixture to the water, along with the garlic (if using).
5. Position your face over the steam and remain there for 5 to 20 minutes. (Bring a handkerchief, your nose will run as your sinuses clear!)
6. Repeat 2 to 3 times per day.

TIP: Similar microbe-clearing benefits can be gained by working with aromatic herbs as incense or a smudge stick (a tightly wrapped bundle of leaves, lit on one end to produce medicinal smoke). A study by Nautiyal et al. in the Journal of Ethnopharmacology found that "[when] using medicinal smoke[,] it is possible to completely eliminate diverse plant and human pathogenic bacteria of the air within confined space." Conifer trees like pine are particularly apt for this.

SINUS-RELIEVING TEA

1 teaspoon echinacea root
1 teaspoon yerba mansa root
1 teaspoon goldenseal root
1 cup boiling water

1. Combine the above herbs.
2. Take two teaspoons of the mixture and cover with the boiling water; steep for 20 to 30 minutes; strain.
3. Take warm, up to one cup per day, as needed.

MUCUS~FREEING TEA

1 teaspoon bayberry root
1 teaspoon white willow bark
2 cups boiling water

1. Combine the above herbs and cover with the boiling water; steep for 15 minutes.
2. Take warm, up to two cups a day.

Sore Throat

Usually, a sore throat is a minor problem that takes care of itself with time. Although we may not always be able to identify the cause of a sore throat, it most often occurs because of viral infections such as the flu or a common cold. It can also occur because of exposure to irritants such as dust or smoke, from allergies, or even from talking or yelling too loudly. A sore throat may make swallowing difficult and may lead to a hoarse voice.

Relevant tissue states: heat (inflammation), dryness or dampness
Relevant herbal actions: anti-inflammatory, antimicrobial, astringent, demulcent, mucous membrane tonic

Herbal Allies

- Balsam Fir
- Bayberry
- Black Elder
- Blue Vervain
- Canadian Fleabane
- Cayenne
- Cinnamon bark
- Coltsfoot
- Comfrey
- Echinacea
- Ginger
- Goldenrod leaf and flower
- Indian Root
- Licorice root
- Marshmallow
- Osha Root
- Sage leaf
- Self-heal leaf and flower
- Seneca Snakeroot
- Slippery Elm
- Sumac
- Wild Cherry
- Witch Hazel
- Yerba sante

Sore throats are generally due to infection, whether that's a simple cold, the flu, or strep throat. When choosing remedies, it is helpful to differentiate between the hot, inflamed, dry sore throat and the cold, wet sore throat induced by post-nasal drip. Use extra demulcents for the former and astringent mucous membrane tonics for the latter. See also Cold and Flu and Immune Support.

SORE THROAT TEA

Makes 2 cups dried herb mix (enough for 12 to 16 quarts of tea)

If you are prone to sore throat in the colder months, make a big batch of this every winter: as soon as you feel a tickle in your throat you can get yourself a hot steaming cup and avoid getting a full-on cold and raspy throat.

Add any spices you like, such as allspice, clove, or star anise. You can also include orange peel: simply chop the peel of your (organic!) oranges and let dry fully before adding.

Stir in some lemon and honey if you like the flavors. Lemon has some antimicrobial action, and the sour and sweet flavors both stimulate the flow of healthy mucus, which fights infection.

You can also add a bit of butter, ghee, or coconut oil: less than ½ teaspoon per cup of hot tea. The medium-chain fatty acids (MCFAs) in these oils are topically antimicrobial and add a nice "coating" quality to the drink.

1 cup marshmallow root
½ cup dried ginger
¼ cup dried cinnamon bark
¼ cup dried licorice root

1.In a small bowl, mix together all the herbs. Store in an airtight container.

2.Make a decoction: Measure 2 to 4 tablespoons of herbs per quart of water and place in a lidded pot over high heat. Add the water and cover the pot. Bring to a boil, reduce the heat, and simmer for 1 hour.

3.To enhance the soothing effects of the mucilaginous herbs in this blend, cool the tea fully after decoction, then continue to cool for 1 to 2 more hours. Strain, and reheat before drinking.

4.Drink liberally throughout the day.

HERBAL GARGLE

Makes 16 fluid ounces (enough for several gargles)

Sage is an aromatic astringent, and it specifically kills rhinovirus: a virus that causes many colds. Combining it with vinegar and salt enhances these properties. If you have a dry sore throat, you may want to follow this with a nice cup of marshmallow tea.

8 fluid ounces water
2 tablespoons dried sage leaf
8 fluid ounces apple cider vinegar
3 teaspoons salt

1.In a small pot over high heat, bring the water to a boil. Remove it from the heat and add the sage. Cover tightly and let infuse for 20 minutes.

2.Strain the liquid into a pint-size mason jar.

3.Add the vinegar and salt, cover the jar, and shake well.

4.Pour off 1 fluid ounce or so and gargle with it for 2 to 3 minutes. Rinse your mouth out with water afterward—the vinegar's acidity can wear down tooth enamel if left in place.

5.Repeat 3 to 5 times per day.

THROAT-SOOTHING TEA

1 teaspoon Canadian fleabane leaves
1 teaspoon slippery elm bark
1 teaspoon echinacea root
2 cups boiling water

1. Combine the herbs in a nonmetallic container and cover with the boiling water; steep for 20 to 30 minutes; strain.
2. Take up to two cups per day, warm.

FRUITY GARGLE

1 tablespoon elderberry fruit juice
1 tablespoon sumac extract
1 teaspoon echinacea root extract

1. Combine the above ingredients and gargle, as needed.

SWEET COUGH DROPS

1 teaspoon goldenrod leaves
1 teaspoon wild cherry bark
1 teaspoon licorice root
1 teaspoon yerba sante leaves
1 teaspoon slippery elm bark
2 cups water
3 cups sugar
3 tablespoons corn syrup

1. Place the above herbs in a pan and cover with the water. Bring the mixture to a boil and boil for 20 minutes.
2. Remove from the heat and cool. Strain the solution and add the sugar and the corn syrup.
3. Place back on the heat, bring to a boil, then reduce heat to medium. Cook until the mixture reaches 300°F (hard-crack stage).
4. Pour the syrup onto a large, buttered baking sheet; cool, then break into one-inch pieces.
5. Use as you would any cough drop.

Sprains and Strains

A sprain occurs when a ligament is severely wrenched, while a strain is a tearing and overstretching of muscle fibers. The same injuries that can cause a sprain can cause a strain as well. The difference is that a sprain involves ligaments and tendons, while a strain involves muscles. Sprains and strains are very common and can cause pain, swelling, bruising, and inflammation. Movement in the affected area is often limited because of the pain and/or swelling.

Most sprains and strains may heal without complications. But more severe injuries can become chronic, develop scar tissue, limit motion, and ultimately cause problems in surrounding tissues, nerves, vessels, and organs.

Relevant tissue states: heat (inflammation), tension and/or laxity
Relevant herbal actions: anti-inflammatory, circulatory stimulant, connective tissue lubricant, lymphatic, nerve tropho-restorative, vulnerary

Herbal Allies

- Big Sagebrush
- Bilberry
- Black Cohosh
- Black Currant
- Cinnamon essential oil
- Gingko Biloba
- Ginger
- Ginseng
- Goldenrod leaf and flower
- Gotu Kola
- Horsetail
- Kelp
- Licorice
- Marshmallow
- Meadowsweet flower
- Peppermint essential oil
- Raspberry
- Self-heal leaf and flower
- Solomon's seal root
- St. John's wort leaf and flower
- Valerian
- White willow
- Wintergreen
- Yerba Mansa

The pain of an injured joint is your body speaking a warning to you. Heed it! Don't let a minor strain become a serious sprain. Rest the joint—but don't immobilize it; gentle movement allows blood to move through the injury site and speeds healing. Drink some bone broth (see Build-Up Broth), eat some seaweed, and work with herbs to reduce inflammation, improve blood exchange, and restore the connective tissues (tendons, ligaments, fascia).

One of the best methods for healing a sprain is alternating hot and cold compresses or baths. Heat exposure brings in fresh blood, while cold constricts the vessels and squeezes out stuck fluids. Alternate between 3 minutes of hot and 30 seconds of cold. Go back and forth a few times, and always finish with hot to bring fresh, healthy circulation to the area.

SOFT TISSUE INJURY LINIMENT

Makes about 8 fluid ounces (100+ applications, 30-day supply)

3 fluid ounces ginger-infused oil
2 fluid ounces Solomon's seal-infused oil or tincture of Solomon's seal
1 fluid ounce tincture of St. John's wort
1 fluid ounce tincture of self-heal
1 fluid ounce tincture of meadowsweet
40 drops peppermint essential oil
40 drops cinnamon essential oil

1.In a small bottle, combine the infused oils, tinctures, and essential oils. Cap the bottle and label it, including Shake well before each use.
2.Hold your palm over the bottle's mouth and tilt to deposit a small amount in your palm. Rub between your hands to warm the treatment, then apply to the painful joints.
3.Massage the oil into the joints until your hands no longer feel oily. Really work the liniment into the tissue.
4.Repeat the application 3 to 5 times per day. More is better!

TOPICAL PAIN RELIEF

20 drops yerba mansa tincture
4 ounces wintergreen oil
1 pound petroleum jelly

1. Thoroughly mix the above herbs with the petroleum jelly.
2. Use as an ointment to relieve muscle pain.

QUICK~ACTING PAIN RELIEF TEA

2 teaspoons black cohosh root
1 tablespoon ginseng root
2 cups water

1. Place the above herbs in a pan and cover with the water; bring to a boil; reduce heat and simmer for 30 minutes; cool and strain.
2. Take two to three tablespoons, up to six times a day.

SWEET RELIEF TEA

1 tablespoon raspberry leaves
1 teaspoon white willow bark
2 cups boiling water

1. Combine the above herbs and cover with the boiling water; steep for 30 minutes; strain.
2. Take as needed.

Stress

Increased heart rate, elevated blood pressure, muscle tension, irritability, depression, stomachache, and indigestion are all signs of stress. To many people, stress means emotional stress. But stress can also be physical (such as the injuries that occur because of a car accident or surgery) and biochemical (including exposure to pesticides or pollution and even poor nutrition). These (and other causes) make the body produce increased amounts of adrenaline. This is how the body copes with stress. But the adrenaline release also causes the heart rate to increase, blood pressure to rise, and muscles to tense.

A host of conditions can develop when the body is subjected to prolonged stress. These include an increased rate of aging, reduced resistance to infection, weakened immune function (which, in turn, can lead to other conditions such as chronic fatigue syndrome), and hormone overproduction (which can lead to adrenal fatigue).
The best tool to fight off the effects of stress is a well-balanced diet and lifestyle.

Relevant tissue states: heat (agitation), tension
Relevant herbal actions: adaptogen, nervine, relaxant, sedative

Herbal Allies

- Ashwagandha root
- Betony leaf and flower
- Catnip leaf and flower
- Chamomile flower
- Elderflower
- Ginger
- Goldenrod leaf and flower
- Hops
- Kava Kava
- Linden leaf and flower
- Peppermint
- Pleurisy
- Rose
- Sage leaf
- Skullcap
- St. John's wort leaf and flower
- Tulsi leaf
- Valerian

Everyone's stress is the same, and everyone's stress is different. We all have the same physiological response to stress—racing heart, shallow breathing, narrowed focus, heightened cortisol and blood sugar. But we react to potential stressors differently—something that bothers one person might roll right off another's back. Whatever is stressing you, herbs can help both as a short-term rescue in the immediate moment and in the long-term to build more "nerve reserve" and poise in the face of difficulties.

RESCUE ELIXIR

Makes 5 fluid ounces (40 to 80 doses)

When you need a quick respite from a hectic day, this is your best friend. This remedy works best if you can step away to a private space for a moment. Center yourself, breathe deeply for a few breaths, take your tincture, breathe a few more times, and return to the world. A little ritual goes a long way!

1 fluid ounce tincture of tulsi
1 fluid ounce tincture of betony
½ fluid ounce tincture of catnip
½ fluid ounce tincture of chamomile
½ fluid ounce tincture of elderflower
½ fluid ounce tincture of rose
¼ fluid ounce tincture of goldenrod
¼ fluid ounce tincture of sage
½ fluid ounce honey

1. In a small bottle, combine the tinctures and honey. Cap the bottle and label it.
2. Take 2 to 4 drops whenever needed.

SOOTHE UP! TEA

Makes 3¾ cups dried herb mix (enough for 22 to 30 quarts of tea)
This is the perfect mixture for those days when you feel like everything is falling down all around you: just take a moment, make a cup, drink it as deliberately as you can, and let the warmth and relaxation move through you.
If your stress manifests with a feeling of heaviness and downtrodden exhaustion, include ¼ cup of dried goldenrod and/or sage.
If it shows up as digestive upsets, include ¼ cup of dried chamomile and/or catnip.
Drink a quart or more every day.

1 cup dried betony leaf and flower
1 cup dried tulsi leaf
½ cup dried linden leaf and flower
½ cup dried rose petals
½ cup dried elderflower
¼ cup dried St. John's wort leaf and flower (see Tip)

1. In a medium bowl, mix together all the herbs. Store in an airtight container.
2. Make a hot infusion: Prepare a kettle of boiling water. Measure 2 to 3 tablespoons of herbs per quart of water and place in a mason jar or French press. Pour in the boiling water, cover, and steep for 20 minutes or until cool enough to drink.

TIP: Omit the St. John's wort if you are concurrently taking pharmaceuticals.

NERVE~SOOTHING TEA

1 teaspoon betony leaves
1 teaspoon kava kava root
1 teaspoon hops
1 teaspoon dried skullcap
1 cup boiling water
1. Combine the above herbs in a nonmetallic container.
2. Put two teaspoons of the mixture in another such container and cover with the boiling water; steep for 30 minutes; cool and strain.
3. Take one tablespoon at a time, as needed.

CALM DOWN TEA

1 teaspoon powdered ginger
1 teaspoon powdered valerian root
1 teaspoon powdered pleurisy root
2 cups boiling water

1. Combine the above herbs in a nonmetallic container and cover with the boiling water; steep for 30 minutes; cool and strain.
2. Take one tablespoon at a time, as needed, up to two cups a day.

SHAKE~IT~OFF TEA

1 to 2 teaspoons peppermint leaves
1 teaspoon valerian root
1 cup boiling water

1. Combine the above ingredients and cover with the boiling water; steep for 20 to 30 minutes; strain.
2. Drink up to one cup per day, as needed.

Wounds

Most wounds are caused by cuts, abrasions, or other physical injuries. Wounds should always be cleaned thoroughly to avoid an infection. The bleeding that often accompanies a wound can usually be stopped by applying pressure to the wound. Excessive bleeding, or injury to major arteries, requires immediate emergency medical care. If a wound turns red, swells, throbs, or is hot to the touch and contains pus, it is a sign of infection: please contact a medical professional immediately in this case.

Relevant tissue states: heat (inflammation)
Relevant herbal actions: antimicrobial, astringent, emollient, lymphatic, vulnerary

Herbal Allies

- Calendula flower
- Chamomile flower
- Goldenrod leaf and flower
- Kelp
- Marshmallow
- Pine
- Plantain leaf
- Rose
- Self-heal leaf and flower
- St. John's wort leaf and flower
- Yarrow leaf and flower

When working with a cut, scrape, abrasion, or other open wound, it's important to always follow the same order of operations:

Stop the bleeding. Direct application of pressure is usually the best way to accomplish this.

Clean the wound. Any particulate or foreign matter must be completely washed out of the wound or it will slow healing and allow infection to take root. A wound wash or soak with astringent, antimicrobial herbs is very effective for this stage.

Prevent or manage infection. Wound washes and soaks are also good here. Herb-infused honeys are extremely effective for this stage, serving both to disinfect and encourage healing. (Don't put tinctures directly into wounds unless you have no other option; even then, dilute them at 1 part tincture to 5 parts purified water, because alcohol inhibits cell growth.)

Encourage healing. Herb-infused honeys, poultices, compresses, and baths are all appropriate for open wounds. Once the wound closes (or if it was never very deep to begin with), you can transition to a salve. Choose herbs that are vulnerary, lymphatic (to drain blisters), and—especially in later stages—softening or emollient (to prevent scarring).

WOUND WASH

Makes 3 cups dried herb mix (enough for 10 to 20 quarts of wound wash)

If you're in a hurry, a simple wash with rose water or nonalcoholic witch hazel extract is very effective during the cleaning stage. After that, transition to soaks and compresses with a formula like this. In the later stages of wound healing, you may want to add ½ cup dried marshmallow or kelp for their emollient effects.

½ cup dried calendula flower
½ cup dried plantain leaf
½ cup dried rose petals
½ cup dried goldenrod leaf and flower
¼ cup dried chamomile flower
¼ cup dried self-heal leaf and flower
¼ cup dried St. John's wort leaf and flower
¼ cup dried yarrow leaf and flower
Salt, for the infusion

1. In a medium bowl, mix together all the herbs. Store in an airtight container.
2. Make a hot infusion: Prepare a kettle of boiling water. Measure 4 to 6 tablespoons of herbs per quart of water and place in a mason jar or French press. Pour in the boiling water, cover, and steep for 20 minutes or until cool.
3. Stir in 1 teaspoon of salt for each quart of infusion you've made.
4. Soak the wounded part, or apply a compress over the affected area.
5. Repeat as frequently as you can, at least 3 times per day.

PINE RESIN SALVE

Makes 8 ounces (40-day supply)

Pine resin salve is the best choice for wounds that have closed or were never very deep. You can work with the resin of other conifers, too. Resin can be harvested directly from the trees—you'll find whitish globs of it along the trunk where branches were lost. Leave enough on the tree to keep the wound sealed—this resin is how the tree forms a scab!
It will probably have bits of bark, dirt, insect parts, etc., stuck in it—don't worry: you'll filter that out during processing.
After gathering resin, use a bit of oil to wash your hands—soap and water won't work. Just drop a bit of any liquid oil you have handy into your hands and scrub as if it were soap. The resin will soften and separate from your skin. Then you can use soap and hot water to wash it away.
You can use plain oil for infusing your resin but starting with an herb-infused oil means you get the good actions of all these herbs, instead of just those the resin contributes.

6 to 8 ounces pine resin or another conifer resin
8 fluid ounces total calendula-infused oil, goldenrod-infused oil, and/or plantain-infused oil
1 ounce beeswax, chopped or grated, plus more as needed

1. In a small pan over low heat, combine the resin and infused oil and heat gently, stirring frequently. The resin will soften and dissolve, infusing the oil with its virtues.
2. Pour this warm oil through a few layers of cheesecloth. Wrap the mass that remains and squeeze it to extract as much oil as possible.
3. Prepare a salve using this resin-infused oil (see here for complete instructions).
4. Apply to the wound several times a day, using fresh, neat bandages each time.

TOPICAL APPLICATION FOR ABRASIONS

1 teaspoon white pine inner bark
1 teaspoon wild cherry bark
1 teaspoon wild plum root
2 cups water

1. Combine the above herbs in a pan and cover with the water.
2. Bring to a boil and boil until the bark and roots are soft.
3. Cool and strain.
4. To use, soak a clean (preferably sterilized) cloth in the solution and apply to the affected area.

TOPICAL WASH FOR CUTS

1 teaspoon pleurisy root
1 teaspoon ginseng root
2 cups water

1. Combine the above herbs in a pan and cover with the water; bring to a boil and boil for 20 to 30 minutes; strain.
2. Apply topically, as needed.

Conclusion

I hope you have enjoyed reading this book as much as I've enjoyed writing it, and I hope it will accompany you in your ongoing journey to the discovery of Native American herbs and their medicinal uses.

If you found this book useful and are feeling generous, please take the time to leave a short review on Amazon so that other may enjoy this guide as well.

I leave you with good wishes and hopefully a better knowledge of the plants around us and their amazing powers.

Printed in Great Britain
by Amazon

68649934R00061